CRY OF OUR HEARTS

A Christian Weight-Loss Devotional

CRY OF OUR HEARTS
A Christian Weight-Loss Devotional

Original material Copyright 2021
by Áccent on Words Press
ISBN 978-1-7342605-2-6
Library of Congress Control Number: 2021911814

Printed in the United States of America
by Ingram Content Group. First Printing

Published by Áccent on Words Press
18543 Devonshire Street #327
Northridge, California 91324
accentonwords.com

Cover photo by Deborah Jackson.
Cover design and copy by Deborah Jackson.
Edited by Deborah Jackson.

Unless otherwise noted, all scriptures are taken from the New International Version. All prayers are considered to be in Jesus' name.

Published in the United States, Canada, Europe
the United Kingdom, Australia, and New Zealand.

Address all queries to
Áccent on Words Press
18543 Devonshire Street #327
Northridge, California 91324

CRY OF OUR HEARTS

A Christian Weight-Loss Devotional

Deborah Jackson

Nancy Urban

Áccent on Words Press

In Memoriam

For Kathy

who is waiting in heaven
for our next get-together.
See you soon.

CONTRIBUTORS

Willie Belt, Pennsylvania, USA
Audrey Bowling, Ohio, USA
Delores Fischer, Missouri, USA
Staci Greunke, Nebraska, USA
Deborah (Debbie) Jackson, Washington, USA
Kathleen (Kathy) Jefferson, Kansas, USA
Sue Lane, Kansas, USA
Patti McCoy, Montana, USA
Vivien (Viv) Moore, South Island, New Zealand
Stacey Nissley, Virginia, USA
Marilyn Nixon, North Island, New Zealand
Pastor Chris Peppler, South Everett Foursquare Church, USA
Nancy Urban, Minnesota, USA
Ria Wharrie, Ontario, Canada

Cover Photo and Design by
Deborah Jackson

Edited by
Deborah Jackson

ACKNOWLEDGMENTS

NANCY: I would like to thank God for all he has shown me and for all his help in writing this devotional.

I would also like to thank my mom and my grandma Wilma for having my back with all their prayers through the years. My mom has always been there for me, encouraging me and praying for me my whole life. She has been my rock.

I would also like to thank my husband, Kevin, for supporting me in the ups and downs of this life. And I so appreciate the many friends who have encouraged me to put the words that God has given me or shown me into writing. And Debbie especially for having faith in me to do this project with her. I have learned much and grown through this process.

DEBBIE: I would like to thank God for his inspiration to do this book and the experience he provided in order to accomplish it. I'd also like to thank my family, especially my mom, Barbara, and my daughter, Jasmine, for their patience with me as I spent so much time writing, editing, formatting, and designing. I would also like to thank Jasmine for allowing me to photograph her beautiful hands for the cover image.

I'd like to express my appreciation to my church pastor, Chris Peppler, for allowing me to use one of his weekly communiques as a post in this book and for being such an inspiration to me with his weekly messages and his constant example of service to our community and to the people of our church.

Finally, I'd like to thank my friend, Nancy. I noticed a long time ago that you have a way with words and that you truly have a heart for God; that's why I knew we could do this together. Even though we've never met face-to-face, you've been my sister in the Lord for many years, for which I'm deeply grateful. Thanks for the prayers you've offered whenever I asked and for all your hard work writing. My goal is to travel to Minnesota to see you soon. And my hope for you is that you'll be able come here to see the Pacific Ocean with me.

Together, Nancy and Debbie would like to thank the ladies of our online group, who have been such a great support to us through the years: Julie Baucom, Willie Belt, Audrey Bowling, Delores Fischer, Staci Greunke, Sue Lane, Patti McCoy, Viv Moore, Stacey Nissley, Marilyn Nixon, Donna Wells, and Ria Wharrie. We'd also like to thank Steve Jefferson, Kathy's husband, for being there to let us know what happened when we had to say goodbye to our friend (for a little while). We would also like to express appreciation to all the other ladies who touched our lives through our little group through the years. We thank God for the awesome gift of friendship.

CONTENTS

NOTE: *Though the principles of the twelve steps and twelve-step programs are mentioned throughout this devotional and are considered beneficial and sometimes vital to seeking a healthy body weight, this book is not affiliated with any twelve-step program. Not everyone who has contributed to this book belongs to or attends such a program.*

INTRODUCTION

Who We Are. Sometime in 2001, a pastor's wife hoped to find a likeminded group of Christian ladies—those who were seeking to overcome the besetting problem of obesity that is so prevalent in our culture. So she did what most twenty-first century women would do, she searched online. When she didn't find what she was looking for, she created her own group. She thought of it as a ministry to others.

That circle of women has seen members come and go over the years; our founder is one who went on to serve in other ministries. And we have moved across three different platforms, communicating first via e-mail and then via social media.

Currently there are fourteen of us. We come from all over the United States, east and west and between, one is Canadian, and two are New Zealanders. Two of us are a set of identical twins. Over the course of twenty years, we have been one another's support system and prayer partners. We have been, above all, friends.

Together, we have experienced the full array of life's joys and sorrows. Along with happy occasions like weddings, births (mainly of grandchildren), new jobs, and moving to new homes, we've been through separation and divorce, serious illness and surgeries (including weight-loss surgery), chronic illness, disability, the physical and mental illness and addiction of family members, adjusting to homosexual and transgender offspring, the death of a child, the death of a grandchild, the death of a spouse, and the death of one of our members. Some of us have had more success at losing weight than others; yet we have never judged each other, just encouraged.

We have enjoyed knowing each other online so much that we

have had four get-togethers in person. One in Iowa, two in Kansas, and one at eight thousand feet in the Colorado Rockies. There have also been several one-on-one visits among members, traveling from U.S. state to state and Canada. We're all aging, but we hope we can get together again at least once more.

Why a Book? Several of us banded together to contribute to this devotional. A couple of us like writing more than the others, so we have contributed more, but that's because we feel it's our calling. A few others contributed their wisdom and talent, when asked (with one guest post from Debbie's pastor), for which we're grateful.

For the most part, this devotional focuses on what we need to do to succeed at the long-term achievement of a healthy body weight. But not every day focuses exclusively on weight loss. After all, part of losing weight and maintaining it is about living life. Learning to live life as it comes along is also part of this weight-loss and weight-maintenance journey. So even if you only have a little weight to lose, or if you have none at all to lose, you'll find that this book is full of practical, biblically based wisdom.

That wisdom comes from the life experience of multiple generations of Christian women who are daughters, nieces, cousins, aunts, mothers, grandmothers, church leaders and followers, and friends. We have worked as wives and mothers, as insurance agents, teachers, administrative assistants, hairdressers, book editors, preschool assistants, waitresses, and college instructors. Some of us have home-schooled our kids, raised disabled children, stepped in to raise our grandchildren, or have taken care of aging parents. Some of us are retired. All of us are believers in Christ (see the Statement of Faith at the end of this book if you'd like to know what we believe).

The Good News. Our prayer is that what we have learned about life can help you in your everyday experiences, especially as you work toward a healthy body weight. Yet our main reason for sharing these experiences is first to share the good news of Jesus with you, because we have experienced his love and power in our own lives.

What is the good news? Though sin has separated us from God, and though our sin has put us all on the road to hell, Jesus paid the price for that sin so that we could return to fellowship with the Creator of the universe (the one who created and has loved each one of us) and ultimately have eternal life with him.

But why would someone want that kind of relationship with God? Because that's why he made you, to be your friend. Because it means knowing the one who knows you better than you know yourself, who loves you perfectly, and who promises to always be with you, even in the darkest times of your life.

If you're in doubt that you're a sinner, just think about the Ten Commandments. Our society is built upon many of them (paraphrased here): God is the only God so don't worship false gods, don't worship anyone/anything but God, don't do evil in God's name, keep the Sabbath, honor your parents, don't murder, don't commit adultery, don't steal, don't testify falsely about someone, don't yearn for something that's not yours. If you've done any of these things even once (lied? stolen? wanted something that belonged to someone else?), you've sinned.

Because God is perfect, his standard is perfection, and none of us can meet it. Not even someone as good as Mother Teresa was. Yet to have fellowship with him, we must be perfectly without sin, because he demands full justice be paid for all wrongs. He knew that was impossible for us, so he made a way by sending his Son to pay the price in our place. God sent his Son, who is God, to die on a cross as payment for my sin and yours.

There exists a great chasm between us and God because of sin, and through his death on the cross, Jesus bridged the gap. He was

God come to earth and lived a sinless, perfect life. He was the second Adam, making a way for us to become sons and daughters of God, to become part of God's family by doing what Adam could not—saying no to temptation and sin. While he was on earth, Jesus said, "I am the way and the truth and the life. No one comes to the Father except through me." He willingly allowed himself to be killed in the cruelest, most torturous way possible because he loved us. He wanted to save us from eternal torment.

First, you must be convinced that you are a sinner in the eyes of a just and holy God. Then you must acknowledge your sins. You must be willing to do a one-eighty, turning away from those wrongs. The result of choosing otherwise is eternal separation from God.

Pray and ask God to forgive you of your sins, believe that Jesus is the Son of God, that he died and rose from the dead on the third day, and ask him to come into your life and help you live for him, according to his will. Then tell someone. The Bible tells us, "If you declare with your mouth, 'Jesus is Lord,' and believe in your heart that God raised him from the dead, you will be saved. For it is with your heart that you believe and are justified, and it is with your mouth that you profess your faith and are saved" (Romans 10:9–10). That's how you inherit eternal life.

Pastor Steven Furtick of Elevation Church has said, "Jesus met people in their messes, in their realities, in their most desperate moments. He loved them . . . when there was nothing lovable or admirable about them." That is the heart of the gospel. That God first loved us and has made a way out of the mess we're in because of our sin. That's the good news. It's the *best* news.

Yet we have given only a rough outline of this good news. It's so much richer and more exciting than what we can say in a few short sentences here. You can learn more by reading the Bible. A good place to start is with the gospel of John, though the entire Bible, from Genesis to Revelation, points to Jesus and the salvation that is found only in him.

About This Book. This book is a daily devotional, with one page to read each day, each with a scripture, a reading, and a prayer. It's organized along twelve spiritual principles, one for each month: 1. Honesty, 2. Hope, 3. Surrender, 4. Courage, 5. Integrity, 6. Willingness, 7. Humility, 8. Love, 9. Responsibility, 10. Discipline, 11. Awareness, and 12. Service/Support.

The ***cry of our hearts*** has been that the Lord will meet us in our need, helping us to do what we can't do on our own strength as we seek to attain a healthy body weight. The crux of what we're saying in this book is that we must rely on God to help us overcome our human failings, even when it comes to something as basic to life as food.

May the cry of our hearts, as expressed in the words of this book, bring you joy, wisdom, and success in your own weight-loss journey and, ultimately, bring you into a closer relationship with Christ.

And let us consider how we may spur one another on toward
love and good deeds, not giving up meeting together,
as some are in the habit of doing, but encouraging one another
—and all the more as you see the Day approaching.
Hebrews 10:24–25

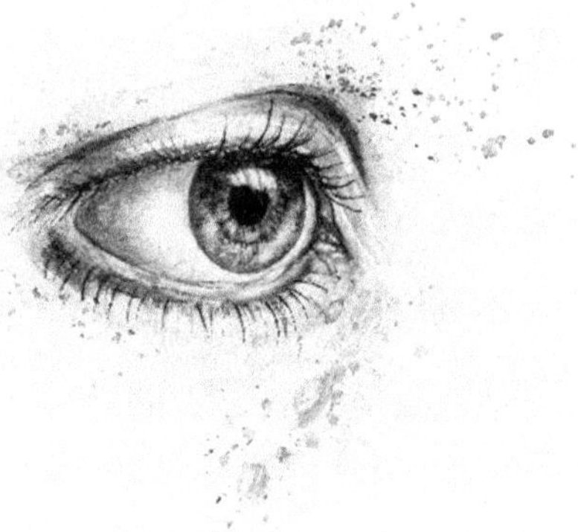

HONESTY

We seek to become honest about our powerlessness and lack of control.

Cry of Our Hearts

January 1

You make known to me the path of life.
Psalm 16:11

The Lord will guide you always; he will satisfy your needs in a sun-scorched land and will strengthen your frame. You will be like a well-watered garden, like a spring whose waters never fail.
Isaiah 58:11

The heart of man plans his way, but the Lord establishes his steps.
Proverbs: 16:9

Enter through the narrow gate. For wide is the gate and broad is the road that leads to destruction, and many enter through it.
Matthew 7:13

If I send a kid to the corner on an errand, she can get from one corner of the block to the other by going straight down the block. Or she can play around along the way, and in so doing go backward around the block or walk three blocks to get to the place I originally sent her. It's the same with your year. You can do what you know you should and make it easier on yourself, or you can choose to ignore what you know works and keep adding on extra pounds. The choice is yours!

Father, thank you for caring enough for me that you even care what I eat and how much I weigh. Show me the way you want me to go, and then help me follow the path you have shown me! Help me not turn to the right or to the left, but help me to stay the course. Help me be honest with myself about my choices and give me motivation when my own fails me. In Jesus' name, amen.

by Audrey

January 2

I have been crucified with Christ and I no longer live, but Christ lives in me.
The life I now live in the body, I live by faith in the Son of God,
who loved me and gave himself for me.
Galatians 2:20

As overeaters, we often don't have an answer for why we overeat. Most of us realize that our emotions often trigger us. But sometimes we're feeling fine and we still eat too much. We don't want to keep living that way. So why do we?

It often doesn't matter that we're believers. In the Christian romance novel *Beyond the Shadows*, the heroine's husband, an alcoholic, recognizes this truth: "Hey, sometimes I'd sit with an open Bible on my lap and ask God to deliver me . . . then I'd lift that bottle and take another drink without blinking an eye. Self-will run amok. But God did deliver me. Not because I deserved it, mind you, but because of his grace and mercy alone. He sent [a friend] at just the right time to show me a way out. He put me in a place where I could face the truth about myself. Admit it and confess it, to him and to others: I'm an alcoholic. I'm sober now. I'm working the steps of AA. I'm depending on God, because I've learned I can't do it without him."

God has led you to this book. You're reading about a way out. Can we confess that we're overeaters? Can we depend on God to deliver us? It's time to take overeating seriously. He wants us to quit lying to ourselves. Why do we think we don't have to be faithful to him in this one area? That is the cry of the Lord's heart for us: Take this seriously! Will you respond today?

Father, help me stop lying to myself. Overeating is stealing the joy and health from my life. Help me to turn my eating over to you today. Amen.

by Nancy

January 3

Therefore, confess your sins to each other and pray for each other so that you may be healed. The prayer of a righteous person is powerful and effective.
James 5:16

Do you know how addiction works? It's like this: When you're addicted to something, your mind gets used to the substance, whatever it is. Eventually, you want a little more and a little more and still more to be satisfied. I can see that pattern with food. Maybe it's not so much my stomach's fault. Maybe my it's my mind demanding more and more.

How do we quit the pattern? It's harder with food. With most substances, you can just give it up. But not with food. So, I believe God honors us if we choose certain types of food to abstain from. Maybe it's chocolate that's your downfall. Maybe you're drinking your calories, and you need to give that up. Maybe it's refined sugar and other refined carbohydrates.

Ask God to help you discover what you must give up to break the addiction. Start with one food and work from there. Then, as your mind wraps itself around the idea that you're no longer going to feed it what it wants, it will stop harassing you.

Once you do that, it helps to be accountable to someone, even better to more than one. And be sure to surround yourself with people who will put it to you straight, those who are willing to stand up to you when you need it. We tend to hide when we're not doing well, so make sure whoever you choose is willing to call you out if she hasn't heard from you in a while.

Father, show us how we need to change our food choices and then help us find people who will hold us accountable, people who are truth-tellers and who care more about our well-being than our opinion. In Jesus' name, amen.

by Nancy

January 4

We all, like sheep, have gone astray, each of us has turned to our own way; and the Lord has laid on him the iniquity of us all.
Isaiah 53:6

There came a time in my weight-loss journey when I recognized that I have no power over my compulsive eating. I have no more power to heal myself from this besetting problem than I do to heal myself of any disease. I wouldn't blame myself for a genetic disorder I was born with. I wouldn't blame myself for having type 1 diabetes or developing some type of cancer. But I have blamed myself for turning to food, for eating compulsively enough that my body became obese. Learning not to blame myself, learning to recognize that I have a disorder, a disease to overcome, frees me to take the *right* kinds of actions. Instead of thinking that my willpower should be sufficient, I instead recognize that I'm powerless, that I have no choice but to seek help.

This realization frees me to see the true answer, which is that I must treat this disease with a three-pronged approach that deals with the physical, the mental, and the spiritual. In the same way that I would turn to a doctor to start the healing process, in the same way that I would begin to apply the correct remedies to heal or manage diabetes or cancer, I must do the same with compulsive eating.

I began with the spiritual by turning my will and my life over to God. I added the mental by being willing to work on the problems in my life that caused my overeating. I added the physical by being willing to change the way I eat.

Father, help me to see the truth about how this all works. And show me the truth about what I need to do to overcome it. In Jesus' name, amen.

by Debbie

January 5

Jesus replied, "Very truly I tell you, everyone who sins is a slave to sin."
John 8:34

I know exactly when my food troubles began. I was carrying my second child, and I had put on a good amount of weight, about forty pounds. Almost seven months into the pregnancy, my son John was stillborn. I went through months of grieving.

At my follow-up appointment, I told my doctor I just couldn't lose the weight. After I had my daughter, I had lost all the "baby" weight within a couple of months, but not this time. The doctor's response was to tell me to take the time to grieve and not to worry about the weight. Something clicked in my head at that moment that gave me the freedom to eat all I wanted. It was after that defining moment that my weight steadily kept climbing.

I'm guessing we all have those moments when we come to a realization that something isn't right. I now realize that my so-called freedom has actually put me in bondage. I now realize that I can no longer give myself that "out." I can't blame my eating on "this" or "that." I can't keep excusing my emotional eating. I have to ask God to break what started way back when and give me the power to say no. No amount of eating will help my grief. No amount of eating will help my sadness. No amount of eating will ease my anger or whatever emotion I'm feeling. But God can!

Father, I pray that when trouble finds me in life, when I'm experiencing pain, that I won't turn to food—but to you. I choose to pray to you, to bow down to you. Please show me whatever it is I need to do to lay it at your feet, to allow you to help me get through my trouble and pain. I'm so glad that I have you in my corner and that you are my comforter. In Jesus' name, amen.

by Nancy

January 6

In you, Lord, I have taken refuge; let me never be put to shame. In your righteousness, rescue me and deliver me; turn your ear to me and save me. Be my rock of refuge, to which I can always go.
Psalm 71:1–3

For the accuser of our brothers and sisters, who accuses them before our God day and night, has been hurled down. They triumphed over him by the blood of the Lamb and by the word of their testimony.
Revelation 12:10–11

Can the fat protect me? Sometimes I feel I'm safe in my own little wall of fat. Nobody can hurt me there. No one would want to hurt me. Coming from a past of abuse I know that has been one of my issues. I felt that if I was fat enough no man would look at me or be interested in me. And then they wouldn't want to hurt me. But life has its problems. The fat can't keep me away from hurt. I was overweight for years, and I had my share of problems. People still managed to hurt me.

The only thing that comes from overeating is more problems. I haven't actually hidden myself under the fat. I haven't protected myself in some shell. I still have to live in an imperfect world. I'll still go through tough times. As much as I want to, I can't hide from my troubles.

But scripture tells us we can overcome them by the blood of the Lamb. God is truly the One who will protect us. He is who will help us through the tough times. And he is the one who will set us free from the bondage of being overweight.

Father, my first instinct is to protect myself from being hurt. Instead, help me to work through the hurts so I don't eat over them. In Jesus' name, amen.

by Nancy

January 7

Therefore, there is now no condemnation for those who are in Christ Jesus.
Romans 8:1

Why is it so hard to think of overeating as an addiction? I think it's because in our society, gluttony is a shameful thing. Let's face it, being fat is looked down upon. We see people who eat too much as weak-willed, weak-minded, and lacking self-discipline. And to even think of overeating as a disease somehow puts shame on us as well.

This used to be true of alcoholism and drug addiction, but not as much now as in the past. If someone admits she has a problem with drugs or alcohol and goes to meetings to overcome it, she isn't shamed nearly as much as someone who carries the addiction in plain view on her body. I think this is because people now understand substance addiction and applaud those who overcome it.

I know members of AA who understand addiction well, but still don't understand the concept of addiction to food. How can you give up something if you still have to partake of it? How can you have an allergy to a substance (as people say they have to alcohol) if you have to put it in your body three times a day?

But it's time to be honest about my problem—it is an addiction, and I must treat it as such. I do have allergies to some kinds of food (mostly refined sugars and other refined carbs) that I do need to avoid. It's time to face the facts. There are some things I have no choice but to stop eating entirely.

Father, help me accept the truth. Teach me that there's no shame in my weakness and show me what I need to do to overcome it. Show me what I need to give up to arrest my addiction to food. In Jesus' name, amen.

by Debbie

January 8

"Woe to me!" I cried. "I am ruined! For I am a man of unclean lips, and I live among a people of unclean lips, and my eyes have seen the King, the Lord Almighty."
Isaiah 6:5

Am I hiding? God called to Adam and Eve, "Where are you?" We all remember that story. We all remember the guilt, the shame they felt after they had sinned. Adam and Eve tried to hide from God, but they couldn't.

If you're like me, how many times have you eaten after the family goes to bed? Or when your family is gone? How much "private" eating do you do? Not to burst your bubble or anything, but it's not so "private." Whether anyone else is around or not, God is right there.

He's watching each spoonful that goes into my mouth. Each fork bite. Each chip. Each scoop of ice cream. Whatever it is that's my weakness. He's watching. It's impossible to hide.

Sometimes I feel that my sin of overeating is so small that I can just put a Band-Aid on it, and all will be well. But it's bigger than that. It's more than just the eating.

Why do I choose to hide behind the bush or tree and then foolishly believe that God can't see me? I cry out for freedom, yet I'm not willing to let it go. I cry, "Lord, here I am." Then I run and hide. I need more than a Band-Aid. I need total and complete healing that can only come from above. I must come out of my hiding place and be willing to be "seen" by the Father.

Father, you see everything, and you love me anyway. Cleanse my heart, my lips, my life. Help me not to hide from you, but instead to seek you freely. In Jesus' name, amen.

by Nancy

January 9

Behold, to obey is better than sacrifice, and to hearken than the fat of rams. For rebellion is as the sin of witchcraft, and stubbornness is as iniquity and idolatry.
1 Samuel 15:22–23 KJV

How many times do I pick up that food that I know I shouldn't have and then stick it in my mouth and eat it? How many times a day do I choose rebellion over obedience? Too many times. I then need to stop and think about rebellion and if I want to continue to walk in it.

A definition of rebellion is: "An act or show of defiance toward an authority." Wow. A show of defiance against God. That's hard to acknowledge, but it's true.

He has set boundaries for us with our eating. He certainly has shown me and told me what I need to do. We all know that junk food isn't the best thing for our bodies. We all know we don't need two plates full of food at one meal. We all know we don't always need between-meal snacks. Yet I show my defiance and stubbornness toward God and do it anyway.

God's word goes even further. It equates rebellion to the sin of witchcraft. When I was younger, I knew some witches. I hung out with them a few times. That was a scary experience. I never want to get close to that again, because there is a real kind of power in it. Which means there is power in my rebellion. I need to knock that power out and take back what I know is right to do. I need to fall on my knees and repent—big time. I need to declare that this is the day that I become rebellion free!

Lord, help me see the truth of the seriousness of my sin. On my knees before you, I repent of the sin of rebellion. Please forgive me. In Jesus' name, amen.

by Nancy

January 10

When Jesus spoke again to the people, he said, "I am the light of the world. Whoever follows me will never walk in darkness, but will have the light of life."
John 8:12

For in him we live and move and have our being.
Acts 17:28

As I write this, it's the summer solstice, the longest day of the year; in some places it's also known as Midsummer's Day. With so much daylight (especially where I am so far north in the Pacific Northwest), it's a good day to reflect on Jesus as the Light of the World. What does light do? It allows us to see the path ahead; it shows us the way. Without light we're blind to everything around us, which means we're also blind to the truth. And without the light of the sun, everything alive on the earth would die. So it is with Jesus, who sustains all of creation.

It's Jesus as the light who shows me things I need to know, such as what kinds of eating I can and can't handle. He showed me a balance between adding to and eliminating certain things from my diet. In doing that, he has helped to remove some of my compulsion to overeat.

He provides the light, the illumination. Once he does that, I have to be willing to see and understand. And if I really want to overcome the compulsion to overeat, I have to do what he shows me to do.

Father, thank you for sending your Son to be the Light of the world. Now that you've shown me the right path, give me the strength to keep going as I take step after step in the way you want me to go. In Jesus' name, amen.

by Debbie

January 11

Finally, brethren, whatsoever things are true, whatsoever things are honest, whatsoever things are just, whatsoever things are pure, whatsoever things are lovely, whatsoever things are of good report; if there be any virtue, and if there be any praise, think on these things.
Philippians 4:8 KJV

What are the things we think on regularly when we're overweight? How we failed at the latest diet? How ugly we look? How disgusted with ourselves we are?

According to Philippians, we are not to think on those things. We're to think on the truth. About pure and lovely things. About things of good report, virtue, and whatever is praiseworthy.

So what is truth? The truth is God's word. And his word says that we're special. We're children of the King. He sees us as the apple of his eye. Like the rose of Sharon.

What is honesty? We can think many negative things of ourselves. But where do we think those thoughts came from? Satan would love to destroy us with our own minds. So being honest must be whatever God says is the truth about us. And we need to quit allowing the lies to saturate our thinking.

What does it mean to be just? It means to be consistent in doing what is morally right. So we think about what is right.

What else does the Lord want us to be thinking about? Those days when we've been successful? The things he has led us to do when we've experienced a weight-loss victory?

Father, help me think about the good rather than the bad, the defeats, or the failures. Help me remember the ways you're leading me into victory. Teach me your truths. In Jesus' name, amen.

by Nancy

January 12

But encourage one another every day, as long as it is still called "today," so that none of you will be hardened by the deceitfulness of sin.
Hebrews 3:13

I read a statement that sent me into a tailspin: "When you justify a weak area, you're in self-deception. And like Judas, you're robbing from yourself."

How many times have I justified my overeating? It's the holidays. It's my kid's birthday. It's my birthday, don't I deserve a treat? It's Easter, Christmas, Valentine's Day, graduation, Best Friends Day. The church picnic or potluck.

I could come up with an excuse for each day of my life. In fact, I think I've done that for more than ten years. Could that be why I've struggled to get the weight off? Could it be the self-deception? When I do that, I'm only robbing myself. I'm no better than Judas. I've only deceived myself, only hurt myself.

Many times I've said to myself, "I'll start fresh in a few weeks." I've even heard people suggest setting a date and then making a fresh start on that day. But I don't think God gives us permission to sin for a few weeks until our start date.

Gluttony is a sin. Consistent overeating is a sin. It's sin because God knows it hurts me. It's a sin through which I punish *myself*. God is only looking out for me. He only wants to keep me out of harm's way. If I could look at it as God protecting me instead of something that I "can't do," maybe that would finally get my attention.

Father, help the scales to fall from my eyes. Help me to see the truth of my sin. Help me to stop making excuses. Help me to finally get honest with myself. And then help me to make a start today. In Jesus' name, amen.

by Nancy

January 13

Then you will know the truth, and the truth will set you free.
John 8:32

Sometimes even when I *know* I have a problem, one of the hardest things to do is to admit that I have that problem. I'd rather go happily along until it becomes so painful that I can't ignore it anymore. Why is that? What is it about human nature that makes us want to walk in denial?

Whatever the reason, I finally got sick and tired of being sick and tired. I got tired of being heavy. Tired of feeling ugly and unattractive. Tired of suspecting that people thought less of me or sorry for me. And I got tired of being unhealthy. Of what the extra weight was doing to my body. I recently read something in a book called *Drop the Rock* that very much applies to me:

> *. . . past attempts to meet our needs have failed. It is recognizing that we are truly bodily and mentally different than our fellows. We are real addicts. If you're a* real *addict, you will stop using some day; it's better to be alive when it happens.*

I'd much rather be alive when I stop eating compulsively. I've been abstinent from sugar for nearly two years. I've lost fifty pounds. That's a good start. But I must remember every day that I'm different. I can't go back to doing the same things that got me to where I used to be. To ensure that I can't go back, I must acknowledge the truth. If I do, it will continue to set me free.

Father, let me always remember the truth. Let me never forget where I used to be. Let me never go back. And let me first recognize the truth so it can truly set me free. In Jesus' name, amen.

by Debbie

January 14

The Lord does not look at the things people look at. People look at the outward appearance, but the Lord looks at the heart.
1 Samuel 16:7

Are you hiding behind a wall of fat? Somewhere deep inside you there's a whole other person crying out, wanting to be free. Maybe you feel like you're suffocating behind the extra weight.

I've felt that way. It all starts in the mind. I may have some fat to deal with, but that doesn't constitute who I am. Some of us are trying to hide. We're ashamed of who we've become.

But we look too much at the superficial. We judge others, and we also judge ourselves, based on appearance. But it's all a lie. We can't truly see the person next to us based on how she looks. She may be beautiful. Have on just the right amount of makeup. Or be buff from working out. But that could be her way of hiding some deep pain behind a perfect facade.

I'm so glad that God says he looks at the heart. Because I know that he would not get an accurate account of me by looking at my outside. If we can wrap our brains around the truth, just maybe we can crawl out from behind the fat and understand who we really are. I believe we're truly wonderful people that others would want to know. Some are hiding abuse, some a hurt from long ago, some a hurt that's happening now. Whatever your story, you should be able to reveal your true self. You can always do that with God. And you're worth it.

Father, help us to see ourselves the way you see us. The same way we see the people we love, you love us. No—you love us beyond what we could ever understand. Help us to feel that. Help us to get beyond the shame and live in your love. In Jesus' name, amen.

by Nancy

January 15

But each person is tempted when he is lured and enticed by his own desire. Then desire when it has conceived gives birth to sin, and sin when it is fully grown brings forth death.
James 1:14–15 ESV

I was thinking about my weight. Thinking of all the old words I've said about losing the weight. I got mad at myself, because it's talk talk talk. That's all it is. Empty words.

There's a movie where the mom tells the kids to use their words wisely. I've started saying that to my kids. Now I need to start saying that to myself, because I'm so full of hot air sometimes it even amazes me. The thing I find myself saying again and again is, "I know what I need to do to lose the weight." So, then, why am I not losing it? Evidently, I don't know what to do after all! I could come back with, "I'm just not making myself." Then I don't know what to do to make that happen, do I?

God talks a lot in scripture about the fool and his words. Whew! I don't want to be a fool, so I'd better start using my words wisely. No more empty words.

The truth is that I don't have a clue how to do this. I'm unwise. I'm foolish. I'm powerless. I can't manage the food. I can't manage my life. I need God to help me. I need to ask God what it is that I'm doing—or not doing—that's blocking my victory in the area of food and weight loss.

Father, I need all the help I can get. I have come to the end of myself. I realize now that I've been foolish. I'm still foolish. I keep giving into a sin that I know will kill me sooner than my life is meant to be over. Yet I want to live. I want to overcome. Help me in my distress. In Jesus' name, amen.

by Nancy

January 16

No one who lives in him keeps on sinning. No one who continues to sin has either seen him or known him.
1 John 3:6

I've been contemplating a saying I've been trying to put into practice: "Cravings are not commands." For a very long time that's exactly what they were to me. Anytime I got a craving, even when I should have been done eating for the day, even when my stomach was already full, even when I wanted a food that wasn't healthy for me, I treated those cravings, those urges as if they were a command to follow. And I gave into them.

Then the Lord gave me an analogy: Photography is a fun hobby for me, and part of it has been to capture pictures of the critters that have visited the forested hill behind our home. Besides the typical bees, dragonflies, crows, and squirrels, I've taken photos of Stellar's jays, northern flickers, a racoon, and two black-tailed deer. I've also heard coyotes yipping and once thought I saw a coyote's bushy tail disappearing into the trees, so I have a desire to take a photo of one.

Problem is, I have a small dog that I let out onto the grassy part of the hill for exercise and to take care of business. Coyotes would be a danger to her, so I need to suppress my wish to see one and pray instead that the coyotes will stay away. The desire to see and photograph one hasn't gone away, but there's a desire that's stronger: that my precious little dog will be safe.

So . . . I need to think of cravings like I do the coyotes. Saying no to myself means protecting some precious things: my health, my character, and my relationship with God.

Father, thank you for showing me the truth. Help me to live it. Amen.

by Debbie

January 17

Do not steal. Do not lie. Do not deceive one another.
Leviticus 19:11

I have fibromyalgia. My body can get so tired that it wears other areas down, so I get pains in areas not typical to the disease. With this disease, I've learned how to put on a false happy face. You could call it a "mask." That's because I feel that no one wants to hear how I'm really doing. So I'll tell people, "I'm fine" even though I feel anything but. I put on an "I'm okay" mask to protect myself. So I won't get hurt by someone's response or lack of response.

It's also true with overeating. I'm not fine. I'm carrying a hundred more pounds than my body should be carrying. I'm putting added stress on my body. But I put a mask on and pretend. I call myself names, but I tell people I'm fine. That's not normal. That's not healthy. And God doesn't want me to do that.

So then how can I be honest with people without pouring out my whole life story? Without sounding like a whiner? That's the balance I need. I need to be able to be honest with people.

One way would be to say, "I'm struggling with an area of my life. Would you please pray?" God's word says he doesn't want us to lie to or deceive others. How easy has it become to deceive people? I don't want to think of it that way, but if I get to the heart of the matter, I'm not only deceiving others but myself as well. I must be honest with myself and God. He's just waiting for me to go to him. He has so much good for me if only I'll ask.

Lord, show me where I'm wearing a mask. My masks can be so dark and carry so much hurt, but you, Lord, you are light. You give all of us the hope of a future that only you can provide. Help me take off my masks. In Jesus' name, amen.

by Nancy

January 18

The heart is deceitful above all things,
and desperately wicked: who can know it?
Jeremiah 17:9 KJV

There are many competing worldviews. One view prevalent in Western culture says that people are basically good and that if they become troubled, it's due to circumstances or socialization. Another is the biblical worldview, which paints a more realistic picture of human nature. Basically, it says, we're flawed from the outset, and the only way to remedy our shortcomings is to turn to God. It's really important to have the correct view of yourself. If you don't, then you can't and won't apply the correct remedy when things go wrong.

Look at the way our society views being overweight: If we just had enough willpower, if we just ate the right things in the right amounts, we would maintain a normal body weight. Or we could look at it as not being our fault. Our parents didn't teach us good eating habits, and some of us had difficult childhoods. Some were abused and used food to self-medicate.

The socialization view recognizes the problem but doesn't provide a remedy. The biblical view tells us we need God, and that's the view that I have found that helps those who have true addictions—whatever the cause and whatever the substance, including an addiction to food. Once we recognize that there is only one way out, by turning our will and our lives over to the care of God, it's only then that we have true hope.

Father, thank you for meeting us in our weakness. Help us to view ourselves realistically and to turn to you as our only true remedy. In Jesus' name, amen.

by Debbie

January 19

This is the way of an adulterous woman: She eats
and wipes her mouth and says, "I've done nothing wrong."
Proverbs 30:20

How many times have I made excuses for my compulsive eating? How many times have I excused my bad behavior by thinking, "I've done nothing wrong"? It starts off with lies. It seems like they're endless. How many times have I lied to myself? How many times have I told myself it's okay to eat the candy (or whatever it is)? How many times have I lied and told God I'll start tomorrow? Then tomorrow turns into years.

There are so many lies I've told not only to God but to myself. How many times am I going to keep doing the same things and not get any results? I'd really love to shove all this on God and say, "Okay, God, do this for me." But the truth is that it's my choice. It's my decision.

I've come to the realization that my overeating is my problem. It's an addiction, and I'm the only one who can work with God to break it. So what am I going to do with each temptation? I've seen when others gave things up—it was hard at first. But the more times they made the choice to say no, it got a little easier. Is the temptation still there? I'm sure it is. I still go through it myself since giving up soda pop. But each day it gets a bit easier. And eventually the victory does come. If I stop lying to myself and admit that I have a problem, that is the first step toward true victory.

Father, forgive me for not being honest with myself or with you. Help to change that, Lord. Help me to see the truth from now on. And let the truth finally set me free. In Jesus' name, amen.

by Nancy

January 20

Do not be deceived: God cannot be mocked. A man reaps what he sows.
Galatians 6:7

I have learned the truth of Galatians 6:7 the hard way. I've made plenty of mistakes in my life, and I hope I've learned from them. Yet I continue to make mistakes, for which I often suffer the consequences, some small, some severe. If only I could learn from the mistakes of others instead of my own! The good news is that anyone can who's willing to listen to the wisdom of others.

This proves especially true when it comes to compulsive eating and weight loss. Now, it's also true that there's a lot of quackery out there, a lot of misinformation, and a lot of people who are mainly out to make money from your misery. But if you look hard enough, you can find the right knowledge.

Yet the Apostle Paul makes it clear here that if we continue to take wrong actions, we'll reap bad results. This isn't new wisdom, it's ancient. He wrote that two thousand years ago. Moses wrote similar ideas about fifteen hundred years before that. The Old Testament prophets practically shouted it from the rooftops.

So not only do I need to seek out knowledge about the food I should eat, but then I need to start walking in that wisdom. I need to take actions, to put into practice what I've learned. I can learn all kinds of wisdom from others, but if I don't put it into action, then I'm still being foolish.

Have you come to a place where you're sick and tired of being sick and tired? Where food rules you rather than the other way around? If so, it's time to seek knowledge *and* take action.

Father, give me wisdom and then help me to DO what you say. Amen.

by Debbie

January 21

Let your eyes look straight ahead; fix your gaze directly before you. Give careful thought to the paths for your feet and be steadfast in all your ways. Do not turn to the right or the left; keep your foot from evil.
Proverbs 4:25–27

I just cannot figure out why it is so hard for me to change my eating habits. I know I can adjust to change. For example, I love to rearrange my house. I'm constantly painting and creating new things for my home. And I like to do different things. I like waterfalls and water; they are ever changing. Yet I struggle mightily with changing my eating habits. I struggle to get some walking in each week. I have to wonder if it's a form of self-sabotage. Do I need to examine whether there's something that God needs to heal in me? I would *like* to see myself differently. I would like to try new types of clothing. I would like to get a makeover. It's not because I can't handle those things.

Anyone who struggles as I do needs to search for these reasons. When it comes to losing weight, we know there will necessarily be changes in many areas of our lives. Our cooking will be different. Our snacks will be different. Even our relationships will be different.

Is it those kinds of changes that scare me? Or could it be a deep hurt from the past that causes me to use food as a way of protecting myself? I'm okay with the idea that it may take some work to get to my healing, but when I do, I will wholeheartedly embrace whatever God asks me to do.

Father, show me what is keeping me from wanting to change. Show me what I need to work on to find freedom from addiction and bad habits. Thank you, Lord, that you want to help me. In Jesus name, amen.

by Nancy

January 22

I see another law at work in me, waging war against the law of my mind and making me a prisoner of the law of sin at work within me.
Romans 7:23

After trying many, many other diets and programs, the only way I have been able to overcome compulsive overeating is through the twelve steps. One of the things I found the most difficult to accept in that program is the idea that my compulsion to overeat, my addiction to certain foods, is a disease.

It helped to go to Merriam-Webster's dictionary for a definition: "Disease: a condition . . . that impairs normal functioning and is typically manifested by distinguishing signs and symptoms." If I can look at my eating problem as that kind of condition, then I can accept it as a disease.

How do I know? Because both my mind and body respond to food differently from normal-weight people. One thing that happens is that when I eat refined sugar, I want more. And sugar also increases my appetite for everything else. Another is that it takes longer than normal to feel satiated when I've eaten enough food to nourish my body.

There's an advantage to accepting my "disease." I can now admit to myself that I can't eat like "normal" people. Just like an alcoholic must never take the first drink, I must never take the first bite of food made with refined sugar. I must measure out my portions and stop eating, even when my body tells me it wants more.

That actually gives me freedom—the freedom to be honest with myself. The freedom to make another, better choice.

Father, thank you for helping me become honest about what's wrong with me. Now, please help me to overcome it. In Jesus' name, amen.

by Debbie

January 23

If we claim to be without sin, we deceive ourselves and the truth is not in us.
1 John 1:8

I was thinking about why I'm overweight and why I can't lose it. But if I'm going to be truthful, I have to say "won't lose it," because I *can* lose the weight. God has made that clear.

That brought up the idea of laziness. So now I combine the "won't" with the "lazy," and I ask myself: Am I using my weight as a way to be lazy? Are there things that I'm using the weight as an excuse to avoid?

So now comes the being brutally honest with myself. I have to answer yes! Yes, I'm using the extra weight so I can be lazy. I waver about wanting to get a job. I'm not sure I want to do this or that. The weight has become an excuse.

I have to ask myself why I don't want to do those things. Because some days a job sounds wonderful, but on others—no way. So what is causing those feelings? The fear of failure? Yes, I do believe that's what it is. I won't lose weight because I might fail at a job.

I also know God has put a call on my life to speak about my past. So I won't lose weight because of the fear of talking to groups? The truth is that all that fear boils down to laziness. The laziness and fear are intertwined. To untangle it and move forward, I need to get before God, confess my sin, and ask for help.

Father, I want more of you. Spirit of God, rain down on me. Lord, I need more of you. Holy Spirit, come and fill me up. When I sing that in church, help me to actually mean it. Don't let me continue to use excuses to not do what you have for me to do. In Jesus' name, amen.

by Nancy

January 24

This is what the Sovereign Lord says to these bones:
I will make breath enter you, and you will come to life.
Ezekiel 37:5

I write a blog that I post to occasionally (someday I'll do it more often). A fellow blogger liked one of my posts, so I checked out her blog and discovered she's recovering from anorexia. Though the scripture above relates to the rebirth of Israel in the Holy Land, it also has much meaning to her, as at one point she was so thin she was primarily just "skin and bones."

I signed up for her bi-weekly newsletter, because I figured that someone who has such a big problem with food, as she did, even though it's the opposite of my problem and even though she's much younger than I am, has some wisdom to impart.

It's the people who have the most to lose, the hundred-pounders (or more) like me, or the people who are literally starving or purging themselves to death who are most likely to come to a point of complete honesty about the seriousness of their problem with food. And it's only at that point where healing can begin to take place.

It's only when I admit the truth about myself and my actions, my poor choices, the way I'm completely missing the mark of where God wants me to be, the way I'm hurting the people around me by my choices—it's only then that I can repent, make a one-eighty, and go in a new direction. It's only then that I realize that I have no power of my own to change. That I need help. Only then will I ask for help from the One who can truly give it.

Father, help me to come to a place of complete and utter honesty. Convict me. Correct me. When I'm walking the wrong way, show me now. Amen.

by Debbie

January 25

But when he, the Spirit of truth, comes, he will guide you into all the truth. He will not speak on his own; he will speak only what he hears, and he will tell you what is yet to come. He will glorify me because it is from me that he will receive what he will make known to you. All that belongs to the Father is mine. That is why I said the Spirit will receive from me what he will make known to you.
John 16:13–15

How do you I see myself today? Lonely, inadequate, defeated, afraid? The truth of who I am in Christ will set me free. I need to find that truth and let it set me free.

God just wants me with him. Not based on what he can do for me, but he wants me to totally, unconditionally want him.

So, whether it is my weight-loss journey, finances, or life problems it's time for me to get hungry to spend time with him instead of being hungry for the food. And let the rest go! He is completely able to take care of all of it.

I'm so hungry for the Lord. I really am tired of thinking about diets, kids, spouse, finances, or work. I'm tired of all that running in my life and running of my life. From now on I want it to be God.

I'll continue to pray for each situation, but I no longer want my circumstances to overtake me.

Father, help me see the truth and then help me bear it. Let me see the truth about myself, my failings, my life, my fears, and what is holding me back from trying to lose this weight. Make the scales fall from my eyes and get me out of denial and into being honest with myself and with you. Lead me into the truth and help me to stay there. In Jesus' name, amen.

by Nancy

January 26

So Moses made a bronze serpent and set it on a pole. And if a serpent bit anyone, he would look at the bronze serpent and live.
Numbers 21:9 ESV

"Just as Moses lifted up the snake in the wilderness, so the Son of Man must be lifted up, that everyone who believes may have eternal life in him."
John 3:14–15

At first glance, the story of Moses lifting up a bronze snake to save the Israelites is a strange one. The people had been grumbling. What about? Food. After everything that God had done for them (freeing them from slavery, parting the Red Sea) it's pretty natural that God would be angry about their attitude, so he disciplined them by sending venomous snakes. It worked. Their attitude changed.

But why have Moses fashion a snake and lift it up? To remind the people that God's justice can be transformed into a source of life for those who look to God for healing. To remind them that they had no power to save themselves, that their salvation could only come from God. Fifteen hundred years later, Jesus referenced this story in his nighttime conversation with Nicodemus.

This is a profound truth: I can do nothing in and of my own power. I am truly powerless. I can sometimes fool myself into thinking I've got control, but that's an illusion. This is also true about food. If I'm honest with myself, I will admit that only God can heal me from my compulsion to overeat. The wonderful news is that if I ask him, he will.

Father, thank you that you are both just and compassionate. Today, I turn my powerlessness over food to you. Take it. Show me what to do. Heal me and give me the power to do your will today. In Jesus' name, amen.

by Debbie

January 27

That is why I am suffering as I am. Yet this is no cause for shame, because I know whom I have believed, and am convinced that he is able to guard what I have entrusted to him until that day.
2 Timothy 1:12

God wants us—daily—to run to him. He wants us—daily—to talk to Him. He wants us—daily—to know that he has our back. Remember that most of all he just wants *us*. He loves spending time with us. He loves just sitting—sometimes just quietly—with us.

If I spend time with God and just be, there is greatness in that. If I spend time just praising him. Not only running to him when I need things. He wants complete fellowship with me.

This verse says, "I know WHOM I have believed." The Apostle Paul didn't write, "I know *what* I have believed."

I must spend time with God the person, not God the gift-giver. That's because God is sovereign. He's not some genie in a bottle to go to when we have a wish for something. He is our Creator, our Father, and the One who seeks a relationship with us every day. And you know what? I believe 100 percent that deliverance from my weight issue will be there every day. Not just Monday but also on Tuesday, Wednesday, Thursday, Friday, Saturday, and Sunday.

It's my aim to get to know God the person better. I'll see if that makes a difference in all the other things that are happening around me. Or at least a difference in my attitude about them.

Father, help me to see your true character. Help me to see the truth of who you are and what you want from me. In Jesus' name, amen.

by Nancy

January 28

From the end of the earth I will cry to You,
When my heart is overwhelmed;
Lead me to the rock that is higher than I.
Psalm 61:2 NKJV

There are times when I'm overwhelmed by my needs. Sometimes I'm lonely, even though I might be surrounded by other people. No one seems to understand what I'm going through. I'm overwhelmed by my sadness, by my aches and pains, by my circumstances. Whatever it is, I'm just overwhelmed, and I end up reaching for anything that will make me feel better.

So many times, what I reach for is my old standby—something to eat, something that tastes good, any kind of comfort food. But for me, this has become a substitute for God, who says that if I cry out to him, he hears my voice. But how many times have I failed to cry out to him in my need? So many.

The time comes when I must recognize my powerlessness over my feelings, my circumstances, my very life. I'm powerless over it all. And because I'm powerless, I have to turn to the One who does have power. To the One who can meet my needs, the One who can do what I cannot. I can get on my face on the ground, recognizing my need, realizing that it isn't food that I need. I need God. I need Jesus. He is the only one who can truly meet my needs. And he will. But I must humble myself and ask.

Father, help me to recognize my own powerlessness. Rid me of any false pride that tells me I can do it all. I can do nothing without you. In Jesus' name, amen.

by Debbie

January 29

Jesus spoke to the people once more and said, "I am the light of the world.
If you follow me, you won't have to walk in darkness,
because you will have the light that leads to life."
John 8:12

Your word is a lamp to guide my feet and a light for my path.
Psalm 119:105

For once you were full of darkness, but now
you have light from the Lord. So live as people of light!
Ephesians 5:8

Do we want to have light in our lives? Do we want to be able to see the truth? Do we want to rest in his peace? Life can throw us such wrenches that it is hard to follow anything, because to follow something can sometimes lead to pain. It can lead to hurt. But this verse tells us there is light. There is life in following him.

The book of James tells us to quit playing the field. Isn't that what I've been doing? And evidently, I haven't hit rock bottom yet. But I will. I'll get on my knees more. I'll cry out to God in a quiet voice and yell at Satan, "Enough!"

I've played this game too long. It's time to stop.

Father, thank you for your patience with me. If you weren't patient, I would be doomed. Help me see the light. And in seeing the truth, let me then take action to do whatever it takes to end this madness of compulsive eating. In Jesus' name, amen.

January 30

If we deliberately keep on sinning after we have received the knowledge of the truth, no sacrifice for sins is left.
Hebrews 10:26

When are the times that I have the most difficulty keeping myself from overeating? When I want to. It's as simple as that. If I'm willing to do what God wants instead of being willful about what I want, then I'm successful. But if I'm willful, that is, if I think I know better than God, if I want something I know he doesn't want me to have and decide to eat it anyway, then I fail. Every time.

One of the reasons we still sin even after coming to faith in Christ is that God doesn't forfeit our freedom of choice even then. He has given me the dignity of free will, and I can and do still exercise it. When I make choices with my free will that align with God's will, then I'm successful. When I make choices that go against God's will (such as indulging in gluttony) then I fail.

Now, God has shown me that there are certain foods I need to abstain from completely, because they trigger me to overeat. Potato chips, cashews, and anything containing white sugar, are on my "No" list. So if I think I know better, and I indulge in any of those things, then I'm being willful in a way that goes against what God has shown me. I'm being disobedient. I'm hurting myself. And that is sin. And what do we know about sin? There are always consequences. When I sin in that way, the effects are easy to see. My clothes feel tight. The number on the scale goes up. I'm uncomfortable. It's not pretty—or fun—or good.

Father, I want to do your will. Make me honest enough to see my willfulness and give me the willingness and the power to do your will instead. In Jesus' name, amen.

by Debbie

January 31

"Am I only a God nearby," declares the Lord, "and not a God far away? Who can hide in secret places so that I cannot see them?" declares the Lord. "Do not I fill heaven and earth?" declares the Lord.
Jeremiah 23:23–24

Sometimes when I take the time to think about how much of a sin it really is to overeat, it hurts my soul. I think about Adam and Eve. They sinned, and then they tried to hide from God. They hid behind a tree and put on leaves to hide their shame. What are we trying to hide? What are we putting on to try to hide our shame?

Sometimes I try to pretend that all is well in my world. But I know that I live with this "secret" sin that is not so secret. God sees and others see. But I don't want to see. I don't want to face the truth of what I'm doing to myself.

But all I have to do is call out to God and ask for forgiveness. He loves me oh-so-much that when he calls out to me it's not to bring shame. It's to bring freedom from sin. It's God who is calling out to me, wanting to help me.

Sometimes this world is so harsh. It seems that when *people* call out to me, it's only to tell me what I'm doing wrong. But I came to the realization that God is the opposite. When he calls, it's out of love and compassion. He longs to see me have freedom from this addiction.

Father, I pray that I will always feel comfortable enough to come to you with all things. That I won't hide in shame or try to hide my sin from you. Lead me to freedom. To health, mentally and physically. You long to set me free. Lord, make me willing to be set free. Thank you for loving me so much. In Jesus' name, amen.

by Nancy

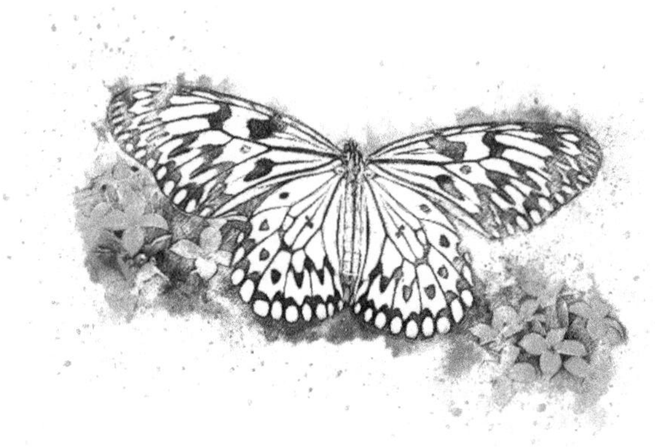

HOPE

We come to understand
that our true hope is in God alone.

Cry of Our Hearts

February 1

Let the wicked abandon his way, and the unrighteous person his thoughts; and let him return to the Lord, and He will have compassion on him, and to our God, for He will abundantly pardon.
Isaiah 55:7

"The definition of insanity is doing the same thing over and over again and expecting a different result." That quote is often attributed to Albert Einstein. It makes sense that such a great thinker would come up with it, but what doesn't make sense is how often I have lived it when it came to food.

Why would I think that I could go on a diet, get frustrated and bored with it, stop, return to my old way of eating, and then expect different results? I did that over and over again in my life. In that way, my thinking about food was insane.

It wasn't until I realized that I had to take a different tack and that I had to do it permanently that I began to have different results. Yet if I had started on that different path thinking it would be "forever," I never would have started. When I did start, it was "just for today." Today I can choose not to eat sugar. And the next day I said the same thing. Until it became a month. Then six months. Then a year. Then two.

One thing that helped was to recognize the insanity of my thinking surrounding food, how I ate, how I reacted to certain kinds of foods, how I hid food, how I had completely lost control. Once I admitted how powerless I was over food, that was the start of being able to turn what I ate over to God. I learned to trust him with my food. And that brought sanity.

Father, thank you for showing me the truth about my crazy thinking and behavior and for showing me a better, saner way. In Jesus' name, Amen.

by Debbie

February 2

For I know the thoughts that I think toward you, says the Lord, thoughts of peace and not of evil, to give you a future and a hope. Then you will call upon Me and go and pray to Me, and I will listen to you. And you will see Me and find Me. When you search for Me with your heart. I will be found by you says the Lord, and I will bring you back from captivity.
Jeremiah 29:11–14

This is my life scripture. It has encouraged me over and over again. When I have felt the most down, that's when the Lord has sent someone to me with this scripture. It's usually someone I don't know, who can't possibly know that it's been a special word to me from the Lord for much of my life.

The thing that stands out to me the most is that God says he'll be found when you search for him with ALL your heart.

Sometimes in life we want to take the easy road. We want to ask someone else to pray for us. We want to leave it on their shoulders. I've done that. I've asked others to pray for me, and then I don't take the time to pray for myself.

Now, we all have times when we're so filled with despair, we aren't able to pray. God understands when it's our friends who must hold us up in prayer. But overeating is different. That's something we need to be on our knees about, asking for God's help and guidance. No matter how long it takes.

God is the only one who knows what's in our deepest being and what is keeping us in bondage. Only he can help us figure it out and work through it. He's the only one who can heal us and break our chains once and for all.

Lord, help me to remember to go to you with my needs. Don't let me get away with excuses. Help me to find my hope and my freedom in you. Amen.

by Nancy

February 3

There, peeping among the cloud-wrack above a dark tor high up in the mountains, Sam saw a white star twinkle for a while. The beauty of it smote his heart, as he looked up out of the forsaken land, and hope returned to him.
J. R. R. Tolkien in The Lord of the Rings

He determines the number of the stars and calls them each by name.
Psalm 147:4

Around twenty years ago, my family and I went through a very bad time of loss. We lost our jobs, our homes, and family members through death. I lost my ability to dream of any future, and I slumped into a deep depression that lasted a long time.

One night as I was lying in bed, I gazed out the window and saw a star twinkling in the night sky. I managed to muster up a prayer of faith and said to God, "Lord, if you could create that tiny star, so far away from me in all its glory, then I believe you can turn my life around again." The months passed, and my fascination grew with what I now called "my star."

Slowly my life began to change for the better, and my mental state began to improve. We moved into a house that our daughter bought, and a few days after we moved, I gazed out of the window and saw my star again, perfectly positioned to shine into my bedroom window as it had in the other house.

Now I get a warm, fuzzy feeling every time I look at it, as it reminds me of God's wonderful saving grace, of his ability to heal. The star is a constant reminder to me that he is fully in control of my life and will never ever leave me or forsake me!

Father, thank you for always providing hope in dark times. Amen.

by Viv

February 4

I am the vine; you are the branches. If you remain in me and I in you,
you will bear much fruit; apart from me you can do nothing.
John 15:5

I once heard sin defined this way: **Sin is people meeting legitimate needs illegitimately**. The truth of that really struck me hard. And it's so true when it comes to overeating and making bad food choices. What am I seeking to do by eating that Big Mac or drinking that calorie-laden hand-scooped chocolate milkshake? I'm trying to meet emotional needs, legitimate ones, but I'm not meeting them in the way the Lord intended them to be met, which is through conscious contact with him. Wow—I really need to work on remembering that.

I know I wasn't normal with my eating. I invariably chose the wrong foods, ate food that wasn't good for me, and—worst of all—ate more than my body needed on a regular basis, which caused me to weigh more than a hundred pounds above a normal body weight. Continually eating in ways that harmed me was a slow form of suicide, though not intentional on my part. But I couldn't help it; every time I tried to overcome it by going on a diet, I failed. Over and over again.

Obsessive thoughts about food are common to people who use food to help them cope with life (me included), but that's not the way God wants me to live. He wants me to turn to him instead of to food. Every time. That's how I meet my needs legitimately.

Father, remind me to ask you for help—when I want to eat when I'm not hungry or when I want to choose all the wrong things—until it becomes second nature to me. You're my only hope. In Jesus' name, amen.

by Debbie

February 5

Look at the birds of the air; they do not sow or reap or store away in barns, and yet your heavenly Father feeds them. Are you not much more valuable than they? Can any one of you by worrying add a single hour to your life?
Matthew 6:26–27

Sometimes I feel like no one really cares. I look around and think that nobody really understands. I feel my weight-loss journey has not been as people seem to think. Maybe they think, "Oh, she must eat a lot." I admit that on some days I do. But on other days I fail because I choose the wrong foods. I don't like to cook, so I've never taken the time to learn how to cook in a healthier way. Learning to cook healthier. Learning to eat less. Those are some of the things I need to do to gain victory with my weight loss. Each is another steppingstone along the way.

When I was young, we went to where the Mississippi meets the Minnesota River. There's an area where you can step on stones in the river and go from one river to the other. It was amazing. So, for me, steppingstones are a positive thing, a step toward a goal. A step toward something amazingly cool.

When I feel like no one cares, the scripture above always comes to mind. God takes good care of those birds. And he says I'm so much more valuable than they are. So I won't worry about the steps. I'll just take them, and God will guide me, because he does care, and he does understand.

Father, help me take each of the steps I need to take to reach my victory. You are my best encourager and cheerleader. You want what's best for me. You say I'm valuable and that worry doesn't help. I lay it all at your feet and then walk the journey with you. Thank you for giving me hope. In Jesus' name, amen.

by Nancy

February 6

But I am like a green olive tree in the house of God.
I trust in the steadfast love of God forever and ever.
I will thank you forever, because you have done it.
Psalm 52:8–9 ESV

After I lost my home and was living in our first rental ever, I was too depressed to look after the gardens. We had a large corner section that everyone could see plainly. As a result, huge thistles grew up, and the flowers were completely choked out by some kind of sticky, clinging weed that grew over everything.

One day, while I was walking to the letterbox, God spoke to me: "Look at this garden. This represents your heart right now, all choked over with weeds. As you start to weed your garden, so the weeds will slowly be pulled from out of your heart."

The next day, I started tackling the weeds. I started with a small section of garden, and when I'd finished, I stood back and looked at it with pleasure. Within a week, I had weeded the whole garden and it looked wonderful! There were flowering shrubs that I had never seen, simply because they were covered in weeds.

I didn't have enough money to buy plants, but some church friends gave me some cuttings. Soon, my garden looked equal to any in the street! I started to care again . . . about things, about life, and about me. I realized, then, that if I don't take care of the small weeds, if I let depression or the cares of this world cause me to despair, they'll end up smothering my life.

Father, thank you for giving me that word that awful day so long ago. Thank you for changing my heart and making me thankful for what you've given me, even when it wasn't what I thought I really wanted. Thank you for replacing my despair with peace and hope. In Jesus' name, amen.

by Viv

February 7

No temptation has overtaken you except what is common to mankind. And God is faithful; he will not let you be tempted beyond what you can bear. But when you are tempted, he will also provide a way out so that you can endure it.
1 Corinthians 10:13

When it comes to food, my problem for most of my life wasn't that I was trying desperately not to give in to temptation, it was that I really wanted to give in. And I did give in, over and over again. Food served a purpose. It comforted me. It meant that I didn't have to deal with uncomfortable emotions, no matter how small those feelings were.

I ate because I was unhappy, frustrated, angry, lonely, bored, or tired, though at the time I didn't realize that's what I was doing. All I knew was that I felt compelled to put something tasty in my mouth. I rarely waited to eat until I was truly hungry. And I almost always chose comfort foods full of sugar and extra fat. Fruit was okay sometimes, but veggies were not my friends.

I wanted to be thin, because overweight girls are looked down on, but I didn't want to give up the things I liked to eat, the foods that comforted me, not even in order to achieve a better-looking body (though the older you get the more health becomes the greater priority).

When being overweight started having health consequences, I knew I needed help. I started attending twelve-step meetings, and through that fellowship and by working the steps I finally found a way to overcome the temptation: by turning to a power greater than myself for strength.

Father, I can't do this alone. Help me overcome this compulsion. Amen.

by Debbie

February 8

The Lord is close to the brokenhearted
and saves those who are crushed in spirit.
Psalm 34:18

I once heard Beth Moore teach that oppression is the feeling of being weighed down in body and mind. Wow! Could oppression actually be the cause of the extra weight on my body?

I was talking with a friend who said she had been struggling mightily through some stuff. As she worked through it, she felt better. She wasn't trying to lose weight, but the next time she went to the doctor, she found that she weighed less. The same thing had happened at other times in her life.

If I don't work through what is weighing heavily on my mind, I'll struggle to get the weight off. Weight loss doesn't just come from choosing to eat better. There are spiritual and emotional components that also must be dealt with.

I need to see why I choose to run to food for comfort instead of to God. Why do I choose food when I'm bored instead of God? Why do I choose food when I'm emotional rather than choosing God?

Beth Moore also said that our prison doors are locked from the inside and that we hold the key. What has us bound there? Something in the past? Something going on now?

I'm the only one who can take that key and unlock whatever is holding me down. I'm the only one who can hold that key out to the Father and say, "Here it is, Lord. Help me!"

Father, today I hold out to you the key to my personal prison. Please unlock it for me and set me free of what has oppressed me for so long. Thank you for giving me hope. In Jesus' name, amen.

by Nancy

February 9

My son, if your heart is wise, then my heart will be glad indeed; my inmost being will rejoice when your lips speak what is right. Do not let your heart envy sinners, but always be zealous for the fear of the Lord. There is surely a future hope for you, and your hope will not be cut off.
Proverbs 23:15–18

We are called to walk in wisdom, but how do we obtain it? I don't know about you, but I have done and said numerous "unwise" things in my life. But if any of you lack wisdom, the Bible says, then ask of it from your Father in heaven, who is pleased to give it to you.

To my regret, one of the unwise things I did was to envy other people. I did that for several years after we had to declare bankruptcy and lost our home. Yet my obsession with what others possessed only magnified my misery.

I had to come to the place of simply knowing that God and God alone was the only possession I needed and that my security didn't lie in things, but in knowing and trusting him. That was a long and painful journey. To the world I was a failure, and statistics show that many bankrupt people commit suicide because they have lost hope. I came very, very close to that point. But God says we DO have a future and a hope, and one day the reward for all our trials will be ours. I long for that great and glorious day!

Eventually, in quite a remarkable way, God gave me (on loan) a home I can call my own. He truly is a great and mighty God!

Father, thank you for giving me hope. Thank you for what you've taught me. Please keep me from living according to my own foolish ways and make me wise as you are wise. In Jesus' name, amen.

by Viv

February 10

As Jesus and his disciples were on their way, he came to a village where a woman named Martha opened her home to him. She had a sister called Mary, who sat at the Lord's feet listening to what he said. But Martha was distracted by all the preparations that had to be made. She came to him and asked, "Lord, don't you care that my sister has left me to do the work by myself? Tell her to help me!" "Martha, Martha," the Lord answered, "you are worried and upset about many things, but few things are needed—or indeed only one. Mary has chosen what is better, and it will not be taken away from her."
Luke 10:38–42

But you, Lord, do not be far from me.
You are my strength; come quickly to help me.
Psalm 22:19

We aren't meant to be everything to everyone or do everything for everyone. Women especially forget that sometimes. Sometimes it's important just to *be*, to fellowship with God and be in his presence. We aren't meant to live the Christian life on our own power, without the help of the Holy Spirit guiding, strengthening, and helping us every step of the way. We can't know what he wants us to do without spending time with him.

Nor can we succeed at overcoming any addiction, including to food, if we don't rely on the Holy Spirit. That's because we are meant to depend on God for our strength and hope.

Father, there are times I know you want me to be like Mary, to choose what is better. Help me to slow down and be with you when you know I need it the most. Help me remember that it's when I'm with you that I can most rely on your strength. In Jesus' name, amen.

by Debbie

February 11

Yours, Lord, is the greatness, the power, the glory, the victory, and the majesty, indeed everything that is in the heavens and on the earth; Yours is the dominion, Lord, and You exalt Yourself as head over all.
1 Chronicles 29:11

Sometimes I need to contemplate who God really is. What he's really like. One way is to think about how big the universe is. It's so huge that we can't comprehend it. It's been estimated that if we were in a spaceship traveling at the speed of light, it would take two hundred thousand years to travel across our Milky Way galaxy. But that's just the beginning. Estimates are that there could be two trillion galaxies in the universe, and the space between them is so vast that we'll never reach across it.

Well, dang. That's one big universe. And an even bigger God who made it. If God can do that, if he can create the universe, if he can create life, then couldn't he help me with something as small—by comparison—as my eating problem?

So, then, do I put God in a box when it comes to what will happen with my weight? Will I choose to limit the blessings he'll pour out on me—because I think he can't help me? Or because I think my sins are too great? How about I take God out of the box? Thank him for forgiving me over and over again. Accept that forgiveness and move on toward freedom with my weight loss. How about if I decide to believe he has the power not only to forgive but to give me the strength to overcome, to walk in victory over my compulsive eating?

Father, you are so much more than anything I could ever comprehend or imagine. Help me to be grateful for your love and for what you said you would do for me. And help me to accept it with gratitude. In Jesus' name, amen.

by Debbie & Nancy

February 12

Let us throw off everything that hinders and the sin that so easily entangles. And let us run with perseverance the race marked out for us.
Hebrews 12:1

Let us not become weary in doing good, for at the proper time we will reap a harvest if we do not give up.
Galatians 6:9

A friend once wrote to our weight-loss group, telling the following story: I once went walking on a trail. On one side was a beautifully manicured golf course, and on the other were dormant farm fields. It was a steady incline, but I kept walking.

Then, at the top of the hill, was a breathtakingly beautiful, serene Amish farm, complete with red barn, white fence, and shimmery silo. It was so peaceful it literally took my breath away.

The Lord used this as a lesson for me and a reminder to me . . . to KEEP going. To not get stuck in rut with the dormant fields. To keep going. Why? Because he'll be there at the top with his prize for me. Keep going. His peace surrounds me. Keep going. His reward for me is waiting for me at the top, but I have to keep going to reach it. It was his reassurance to me that I've traveled a long way on this weight-loss journey, but I haven't reached the end yet. God has a plan for me, but I have to be willing to walk through the ruts, the dormancy, and the hills and accept his plan for me. He knows what's at the top of the hill for me, and if I'm willing to keep walking in his way, he will take my breath away! Praise him!

Father, help me to keep going on the path you have set before me; help me remember that the reward will be better than I can ever imagine. In Jesus' name, amen.

by Teresa & Debbie

February 13

But the one who hears my words and does not put them into practice is like a man who built a house on the ground without a foundation. The moment the torrent struck that house, it collapsed, and its destruction was complete.
Luke 6:49

Have you ever had the Lord shake you up? I had been asking God why it seemed so hard to do the right things on this weight-loss journey. It seemed like I had been doing everything wrong.

I asked God to put the fire back in me. To put that overwhelming desire back. I then realized that my words were not lining up. I was not confessing the positive. In fact, I was whining. I think the Lord had enough of my complaining, because he had a dear friend send me a rough letter. She did not pull any punches. It's no fun getting hit between the eyes, but oh so good, because that meant the victory was coming.

My friend talked about there being no room for discouragement. And you know what? The Lord told me that in the very beginning, that if I kept a positive attitude and confessed positives throughout this journey, I would make it. But if I started talking defeat, I would be defeated.

I've noticed as my words have not lined up, the weight has not come off, and when my words line up, the weight comes off. It's like I used to tell my kids: "The Lord is not going to come to your pity party." Apparently, I needed a reminder.

We all get discouraged sometimes, but there's no room for wallowing in it! Obedience is no small thing! We must be hearers that do!

Father, help me to remember that my peace, my encouragement is in you. And let me not just hear your words, but act on them too. In Jesus' name, amen.

by Nancy

February 14

He has made everything beautiful in its time. He has also set eternity in the human heart; yet no one can fathom what God has done from beginning to end.
Ecclesiastes 3:11

Why is it so much easier for children to believe in God? Is it just because their understanding is so simple? I think it's because they're so much closer to the magical, the supernatural, the eternal. Maybe that's why Jesus told us we must approach God like little children; the very young trust in the eternal. I'll never forget the first time someone told me I would die one day. I was five and had no understanding of death. My grandmother assured me that it would not happen for a long time, that I might live to be a hundred. The same moment happened in my son's life at the same age, but that time I was the one providing the reassurance.

There's something in our nature that makes us want to believe in something bigger than we are, that makes us long for something more than this mundane existence we experience in our everyday lives. Even as adults, there's something in us that longs for magic to be true. A place inside us that hopes for life to last forever. Something that makes our struggles worthwhile, that rewards all our effort, striving, and pain. We have a deep desire to find and experience something magical, because there is a magical Person and a magical place to long for. We yearn to see the future, to live beyond death, and to find true justice, peace, happiness, meaning, and—most of all—love. God put that longing in us, and he is the only one who can satisfy it.

Father, thank you for putting eternity in my soul so that I would have to turn to you to be satisfied by your love. In Jesus' name I pray, amen.

by Debbie

February 15

For you have been my refuge,
a strong tower against the enemy.
Psalm 61:3

We have this hope as an anchor for the soul, firm and secure.
It enters the inner sanctuary behind the curtain.
Hebrews 6:19

How many of us have songs that really speak to us? One of mine is "The Anchor Holds" by Ray Boltz. I have listened to that song through personal trials, and it also became our family song as we went through some challenges. The song talks about rough waters and how an anchor holds. One part says:

I have fallen on my knees and faced the raging sea,
The anchor holds in spite of the storm.

How many times has the Lord, our Anchor, been there for us? For those who have been abused or are going through it now, his anchor holds. He's going to get us through the storm. He'll steady us. He'll make sure that we are not moved away from him. He is anchoring us.

We may seem alone at times. We may think we just can't take any more of what this sea of life tosses our way. We may wonder why we're facing a certain situation, but we have the assurance of his word that God is going to get us through it somehow.

Today, I can allow him to be my Anchor.

Father, you may not always calm the seas, but I know you can calm me in the midst of the storm. Thank you. In Jesus' name, amen.

by Nancy

February 16

Let the words of my mouth and the meditation of my heart be acceptable in your sight, O Lord, my strength and my redeemer.
Psalm 19:14 NKJV

Last year, I finally did what I had been promising myself I would do for a while: I read Rick Warren's *The Purpose Driven Life.* When I was done, I came up with a purpose statement for myself:

God's ultimate purpose for my life is to make me more like Christ. To allow him to do that I must put my complete faith and trust in him in all things. I must give him my talents, my shame, my fears, my hopes, my goals, and my dreams. I must make him my ultimate dream, because I know that it is in him that I will find my ultimate fulfilment. When I stand before him on Judgment Day, my hope is to hear him say, "Well done, my good and faithful servant."

Part of that purpose has been to be obedient to God in all things, including in the types and amounts of food I choose to eat. I'm still a work in progress in that area, and God is continuing to refine both the types and amounts of food I consume. Thank goodness he's so patient with me! The most wonderful thing to come out of this weight-loss and purpose-finding journey has been to feel that I am sitting in the very middle of God's will for my life. That gives me such a sense of peace and joy. It means I can be filled with joy in all circumstances, even the difficult ones. It means I can trust God to always do what's best for me.

Father, my heart is full of gratitude today for all you have done for me. Most of all, thank you for giving me a true sense of purpose, fulfillment, hope, and peace. In Jesus' name, amen.

by Debbie

February 17

Whatever is noble, whatever is right, whatever is pure, whatever is lovely, whatever is admirable—if anything is excellent or praiseworthy—think about such things.
Philippians 4:8

As I write this, I've recently been through lot of sadness, grief, confusion, and discontent. I have needed God to answer a lot of prayers lately. And through it all he's been teaching me. Don't you love how he takes the rough times and uses them as school lessons?

I had already been taught to have faith. But what exactly is faith? The dictionary says it's a confident belief in the truth, belief that doesn't rest on logical proof or material evidence. So how do I get that faith? I pray and receive it. So I have faith, but still no answers to my problems.

Then I've been taught that I have to believe for it. What is belief? The dictionary says it's the mental act of placing trust or confidence in something. So I believe that God is going to come through. I've believed for months now, and still no answer.

So I studied again and saw that I need to expect great things. So what is expectation? The dictionary says it is "To consider it likely. To look forward to something." As of today, I have walked through these three stages, and the Lord reminded me that I am to always think on his ways, think his thoughts. He reminded me that I need to think on what is lovely and pure. To meditate on his promises. And wait in faith, belief, and expectation.

Father, teach me to expect the right things, to expect to do well with my eating. Teach me to walk through the day confident in the truth you've shown me. Teach me to trust you with confidence. Teach me to look forward in expectation of receiving the prize of good health and a beautiful body. Amen.

by Nancy

February 18

My tears have been my food day and night,
while people say to me all day long, "Where is your God?"
Psalm 42:3

A part of any Christian walk is a point when God feels distant. He isn't, but for some reason I have felt that way. In those times, what can I do to cope?

I can trust God's word. I can trust what he said, even though my feelings don't back it up. And yet, that may not always work, either, because not everything I read speaks to me. Perhaps because I'm not ready to hear and absorb it.

In those times, I have to act as if. As if God is near, as if I can trust him, as if he's always ready to help me. Even if I don't feel it. Even if he feels distant. Even if I'm not hearing his voice. I need to always remember that:

Neither death nor life, neither angels nor demons, neither the present
nor the future, nor any powers, neither height nor depth,
nor anything else in all creation, will be able to separate us
from the love of God that is in Christ Jesus our Lord.
Romans 8:38

Father, help me to learn what you want and need me to learn, even when I don't feel your presence. Help me to understand and to do your will even when you seem far away. Help me to be patient as I wait on those things I've prayed about for a long time, and your answer has still been, "Wait." Help me to cling to you even when I feel desolate and lonely. Let your words of hope comfort me always. In Jesus' name, amen.

by Debbie

February 19

I no longer call you servants, because a servant does not know his master's business. Instead, I have called you friends, for everything that I learned from my Father I have made known to you.
John 15:15

And the scripture was fulfilled that says, "Abraham believed God, and it was credited to him as righteousness," and he was called God's friend.
James 2:23

How do you see God? What assumptions do you make about him? Is it at all possible that the way you view God isn't actually who he really is? I willingly grant that for myself. God has corrected my view of him many times.

Once, a stranger came up to me to tell me that God wanted me to know how much he loved me. I thought I already knew that, but that incident caused me to contemplate God's love even more. One of the most important things I had to learn was that God cares about my weight and my struggles with food. And that he is willing and able to help me overcome my constant compulsion to overeat. Does God care about what I eat for breakfast? Does he care that my body responds to sugar like it might to heroin? That I somehow can tolerate eating a few corn chips, but that eating one potato chip means that I won't stop until I've eaten the whole bag?

God cares about all of it, and he's willing and able to help me overcome my addiction to certain foods, to help me overcome my compulsion to overeat. Why? Because the amazing truth is that God, the creator of the universe, is my friend.

Father, help me to see you clearly, so that I'll understand that you want to help me through my struggles with food. In Jesus' name, Amen.

by Debbie

February 20

Those who sow with tears will reap with songs of joy.
Psalm 126:5

I hit a rough patch in my life, and it made me wonder—what is real joy? I've heard preachers who tried to encourage people to find joy in every situation. Yet my heart was breaking. I know they were trying to help. But my brain, my thinking, only brought condemnation, because I started to wonder what was wrong with me that I couldn't find joy in that situation. Did that make the Lord even more upset with me for not finding the joy?

God created us. He put us on this earth, emotions and all, and told us there's a season for everything. Yet I found it hard to find joy when everything around me was at its worst. So I looked up what it means. The dictionary says:

> ***Joy*** *[noun] 1: the emotion evoked by well-being, success, or good fortune or by the prospect of possessing what one desires; 2: a source or cause of delight.*

That tells me that I can have joy in the expectation of having something. There is also a source of that joy. When I have my rough days and I think I just cannot make it one more day, I can still have joy, because the source of it is the Lord and in what I can expect from him. I have that with me every day. I'm thankful I can have pleasure in the company of my Lord, that I can find happiness in him no matter my circumstances.

Father, I know you understand my feelings. Help me not to beat myself up if I'm having a teary, weepy, want-to-give-up day. Thank you for loving me just the way I am, emotions and all. In Jesus' name, amen.

by Nancy

February 21

This is the confidence which we have before Him, that,
if we ask anything according to His will, He hears us.
And if we know that He hears us in whatever we ask, we
know that we have the requests which we have asked from Him.
1 John 5:14–15

And we know that God causes all things to work together for good to
those who love God, to those who are called according to His purpose.
Romans 8:28

My thinking sometimes tells me that some things are impossible, that God just doesn't do them in today's world. Instead, I need to have faith that God can do ANYTHING that's within his will. Even when I'm doubtful, God has the power to provide complete healing, salvation, a change of attitude—all of which sometimes seem impossible in seemingly insurmountable situations. There is a difference between knowing God can do anything and realizing that his answer to prayer today may be yes, wait, or no. That's where trust comes in. It's my job to take my wishes, the prayers I've been praying so earnestly, and trust that no matter what God's answer is, it's in his will for my life or the lives of the people I'm praying for.

Not only that, but whatever God's answer to my prayer is, I can trust that it's in my best interests, that whatever I'm going through will work out for my good.

Father, help me learn to trust you. To have hope in you, like Abraham did. Like David did. Like Jesus did. When you say yes, I'll say thank you. When you say wait, give me patience to keep praying. When you say no, please help me to accept your will as the right thing for me. In Jesus' name, amen.

by Debbie

February 22

"Restrain your voice from weeping and your eyes from tears, for your work will be rewarded," declares the Lord. "They will return from the land of the enemy. So there is hope for your descendants," declares the Lord. "Your children will return to their own land."
Jeremiah 31:16–17

Ask and it will be given to you; seek and you will find; knock and the door will be opened to you. For everyone who asks receives; the one who seeks finds; and to the one who knocks, the door will be opened.
Matthew 7:7–8

Are you the parent of a prodigal? If not, you probably know someone who is. Or maybe you were the prodigal and you have finally returned to the Lord.

Stand strong, Mama. There are many, many of us out there who are or have been the mothers of some very troubled children, sometimes when they're young, and sometimes when they've already been adults for a long time. Often, it's just as they're gaining their independence from us.

Never underestimate the power of a praying mother. Keep praying for your children's safety, for their deliverance, for their healing, and that they will return to the Lord they were taught about when they were young. And if you weren't a believer when you were raising them, you can still pray for them to come to a saving faith.

Father, please encourage us as mothers to continue to pray for our children in faith. Give us hope and let us not grow weary of knocking on heaven's door as we ask you to protect, guide, heal, deliver, and save our children. In Jesus' name, amen.

by Debbie

February 23

But the seed falling on good soil refers to someone who hears the word and understands it. This is the one who produces a crop, yielding a hundred, sixty, or thirty times what was sown.
Matthew 13:23

Now to him who is able to do immeasurably more than all we ask or imagine, according to his power that is at work within us.
Ephesians 3:20

I've been doing a lot of thinking lately about dreams. What dreams I had for my life. What dreams I still have. With the rapes, the loss of children, and a failed marriage, I cast my dreams aside. I felt they were unattainable. It even became hard to figure out what I still dream about. Yet does God want us to dream? He certainly wants us to have hope for the future. I believe he plants dreams in us to get us where we need to go.

I remember some of my smaller dreams—as a Midwest gal I had a dream of seeing the ocean, of wanting to visit inside a lighthouse. But what about the big dreams? What do I want to do with my life? The flip side of dreams is fear. We are so often filled with so many fears. I was praying the other night, and I wanted to say, "Your will be done, Lord." But I couldn't, because it scared me. I admitted to God that I felt nervous about what he might ask me to do. I felt that I couldn't attain whatever it might be.

Then I remembered that it's not about me. God can attain anything if I'm a willing vessel.

Father, make me willing to do your will. Help me step out in faith, no matter what you ask me to do. Help me always have hope in you. Amen.

by Nancy

February 24

For it is God who works in you to will and
to act in order to fulfill his good purpose.
Philippians 2:13

Sometimes the idea of becoming disciplined enough to actually lose weight and keep it off seems overwhelming. So how can I do it without having to just grit my teeth and bear it? Without having to hold on for dear life as if I were hanging over a precipice ready to drop to my death, white knuckles showing from the strain? Well, I certainly can't do it on my own power. I like what Bible teacher Priscilla Shirer wrote about this concept:

> *So relax. Presenting yourself to the Lord is an exercise in gratitude. It's something you can sustain, not by tireless effort, but only by walking in step to the rhythm of His grace and depending on the empowerment of His Spirit. Seek Him in prayer and ask for insight on how He wants you to adjust your life to best honor Him. He will give you the clarity, and He will also give you the desire to please Him.*

That means I don't have to white-knuckle my abstinence from compulsive eating. I can relax and ask God to get me through the cravings, the urges, the tendency to turn to food for comfort (or even just out of habit). God wants me to succeed at this. He's not standing over me, prying open my fingers so I'll let go and fall. If I do fall off the wagon, he wants to pick me up, put me back on, and even bandage the scrapes that resulted when I hit the pavement. So relax! God's got this. He's got *you.*

Father, I believe you can help me succeed at the impossible. Give me your strength. In Jesus' name, amen.

by Debbie

February 25

Then he cried out to the Lord, "Lord my God, have you brought tragedy even on this widow I am staying with, by causing her son to die?" Then he stretched himself out on the boy three times and cried out to the Lord, "Lord my God, let this boy's life return to him!" The Lord heard Elijah's cry, and the boy's life returned to him, and he lived.
1 Kings 17:20–22

One thing I've noticed about the prophet Elijah was that he was audacious. Audacious enough to ask God for big things. Impossible things. Like calling down fire from the sky in front of a huge crowd. Like raising a widow's son from the dead.

God has been showing me is that it's okay to ask big. If there's an impossible problem I'm facing or something he's given me a desire to do that I never thought was possible (because there's not enough money or time), then I should go ahead and ask. So I made a list of impossible things to ask for. Healing and deliverance for family members with mental illness and addiction. Willingness to change my diet again so that I'll continue to lose weight. Healing of my own "thorn in the flesh," my compulsion to overeat. Provision for things I didn't think I could afford.

Though God often uses suffering and difficulties to refine us, he also wants to give good gifts to his children. Sometimes I forget that. There is a caveat, however. To get what Elijah received, I need to be willing to do what Elijah did. Elijah was obedient. He did what God asked, without question. Am I willing to be just as obedient?

Father, help me to be more like Elijah, to obey you when I hear your voice. Yet remind me that you want me to ask for the big, impossible things too. And let me not be afraid to ask for them when it is your will. In Jesus' name, amen.

by Debbie

February 26

He says, "Be still, and know that I am God; I will be exalted among the nations, I will be exalted in the earth."
Psalm 46:10

Dr. Jack Hayford wrote: "Living in a miracle means far more than experiencing its conception. It means resting in God's promise and power even when it seems the miracle isn't going to be born." After I read that, I thought about my dreams. First, I asked myself and then I asked God, "Have I put my dreams ahead of God?"

I think back to all the times I prayed for this or that. I think about all the let-downs after what I prayed for didn't happen. I think of all the anger. Then it dawned on me: I put the dreams ahead of God. If God had been first, why would I be mad at him if he said no? If I totally trusted that God knows exactly what I need and when, then why the anger?

I need to lay down all my dreams. I need to trust that God is fully in control. I don't write my own story; God already has the novel done. Do I want to change it? Or do I want to trust that he is perfectly able to meet all my needs abundantly?

Letting go of my dreams is probably one of the hardest things that I can do. But I know it will be rewarding, because I'll have a deeper relationship with God. Am I saying I shouldn't have dreams? No. But if I do, I need to make sure that God comes before them. I need to be excited to experience God. Then if the dreams happen, all that's left to do is praise him.

Father, I know putting my dreams in your hands doesn't mean giving up hope. But it does mean putting my life in your hands. Help me to trust you enough that I can do that with my future as well as my present. Amen.

by Nancy

February 27

No temptation has overtaken you except what is common to mankind. And God is faithful; he will not let you be tempted beyond what you can bear. But when you are tempted, he will also provide a way out so that you can endure it.
1 Corinthians 10:13

What do you do when you experience the typical irritation and frustration that anyone feels living and working with other human beings? Especially when they aren't doing things the way you believe they should be done?

Even now, I sometimes get a momentary reaction to those feelings that was typical of me in the past—a sudden desire to put something in my mouth and eat. In other words, my negative emotions make me think I'm hungry when I'm not.

If it's not time to eat when that happens, what can I choose to do instead? I can take a contrary action—do something other than what I'm currently doing. Some of the things I've have chosen to do are read God's Word, take a walk, sing a song, take a long drink of water, and—most often—pray and ask God to help me through it. I'm grateful that I have a program that tells me, "This too shall pass." If I wait rather than giving in to the false hunger, it does go away. It sometimes takes longer than at other times, but usually it passes far more quickly than I expect. That gives me hope.

When I have asked for help, Jesus has not failed me. Unhealthy desires for food I don't need become fleeting and weak against the power of an amazing and caring God.

Father, when I ask for help, bring to mind something that I can do that will allow me to wait out the temptation long enough for it to pass. In Jesus' name, amen.

by Debbie

February 28

Let us hold unswervingly to the hope we profess,
for he who promised is faithful.
Hebrews 10:23

He gives strength to the weary and increases the power of the weak.
Isaiah 40:29

It's important to give thanks and praise to God, to worship him not only for what he has done, but for the things that have not yet happened. The things I have been longing for and praying for fervently. As if they had already taken place.

Have I been praying for a family member? For healing? For deliverance? For some problem that has been going on a long time for which I'm awaiting a resolution?

What about reaching a healthy body weight? Overcoming a food obsession and the compulsion to overeat?

I must praise and thank God for the things I've been asking him for. He is a good and faithful Father who only wants my ultimate good. He loves me with an amazing, unfathomable love. He has made many promises, and he has kept them, even though he still has more to keep.

I can wait in hope and trust and with the understanding that he is working toward my ultimate good. I can stand in hopeful expectation of those answers he is so willing to provide.

Thank you, Lord, for my life. Thank you for my mistakes, because without them I would never have learned the lessons you wanted to teach me. Thank you for removing my sins as far as the east is from the west. Thank you for being my strength. Thank you for being a promise keeper. In Jesus' name, amen.

by Debbie

February 29

This is what the Lord says: "Look! I am preparing a disaster for you and devising a plan against you. So turn from your evil ways, each one of you, and reform your ways and your actions." But they will reply, "It's no use. We will continue with our own plans; we will all follow the stubbornness of our evil hearts."
Jeremiah 18:12

Being honest with ourselves can be so hard. We think we have it together. We think we know what's best. We think we're the Holy Grail of sainthood. Those who feel that way are just as bad as "fans" of Christ who aren't really followers of Christ. It's become about themselves. So it's time to be honest. Time to check myself. Keith Green sang a song called "My Eyes Are Dry." Are my eyes dry? The lyrics say: *My faith is old. My heart is hard. My prayers are cold.*

But what causes my heart to be hard? Exploring the answer to that might open a whole can of worms. Is it because of something that happened that I'm bitter about? Is it because of a trauma that makes it hard for me to trust anyone? Or am I judging someone else who's having a hard time softening his heart? I think if we're honest, everyone can say, "My heart is hard." To some extent. But the good news is that God says he can fix that: *I will give you a new heart and put a new spirit in you; I will remove from you your heart of stone and give you a heart of flesh* (Ezekiel 36:26).

Father, thank you for giving me hope that you can finally change me. That you can take the sin that I've been practicing for years, an addiction that's overwhelming, and you can help me walk out of it for good. In Jesus' name, amen.

by Nancy

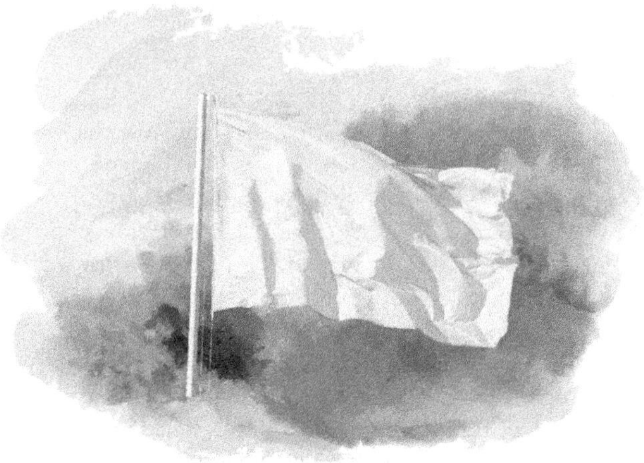

SURRENDER

We discover that surrendering to God is the only way.

CRY OF OUR HEARTS

March 1

Take my life, a sacrifice; In You alone I'm satisfied
Here I empty myself to owe this world; Nothing and find everything in You
Not my will, but Yours be done; Not my strength, but Yours alone
Nothing else, but You oh Lord; I surrender all to You
I Surrender *by All Sons & Daughters*

My son, give me your heart, and let your eyes observe my ways.
Proverbs 23:26

Many reading this book already understand the idea of surrender, because you've done it. You gave your heart and your life to Christ and became a believer. He has changed you and your life. And yet you still struggle with food. It seems to own you. Your weight is out of control. It's affecting your health and happiness. You're tired of being heavy. You're tired of being sick and tired. If so, you may already recognize that it's time to make another surrender. This time you'll be surrendering your food to God. The fact that you have picked up this book to read it, I'm assuming with the hope that it will help you learn how to lose weight, tells me that you've already begun the process of surrender. Don't take that lightly. It means something. You've begun to open the door. Perhaps now you can walk through it.

Don't be afraid to surrender your food, because what I discovered after doing it is that it brought me freedom. It has allowed me to give away fifty pounds that I'm now free of—I hope forever. God loves you and can give you the strength to do what you cannot do without him. It's always the right time to walk through that door. It's always the right time to surrender.

Father, I surrender all to you. Including my food. In Jesus' name, amen.

by Debbie

March 2

Call on me in the day of trouble; I will deliver you.
Psalm 50:15

What did it take to lose fifty pounds in a year? How did I walk through that door, and what will keep me from going back to the awfulness of being that heavy?

Surrender is the hinge on which the door rests. Surrender is the willingness to say to God, "I give up. I can't do this on my own strength. I need you to help me. I'll do whatever you want me to do. Just let me know what that is. Yet, help me, Lord, because I can't do it under my own power. If you want me to accomplish it, you'll have to help me all along the way."

Anyone who wants to walk through the door that overcomes an addiction—no matter the substance, including food—must have that hinge on their door. Otherwise, the door simply won't open. Think about how hard it is to open a door with rusty or broken hinges. You're working so hard on your own power to try to open that door. You might be able to pry it open just enough to squeeze a finger or even a hand through, but it will never open all the way.

Father, please help me to make you truly the Lord of my life. Help me to let go of those things I'm clinging to so desperately that are holding me back. Help me to place a well-oiled, functioning hinge on the door I know you want me to walk through. I know I must acknowledge my sin, ask you to remove it, and turn my will and my life over to you. Please take me and help me to live according to your will. Whatever you ask, Lord, I'm willing to do it, no matter what it is. Please help me to do your will, minute by minute, because I can't do that in my own power and strength. In Jesus' name, amen.

by Debbie

March 3

Come near to God and He will come near to You. Wash your hands, you sinners, and purify your hearts, you double minded.
James 4:8

I just can't do this myself. I've tried. I've thought I could do it myself. I've thought, "You've made your bed now lie in it." I've felt that because I did this to myself, why would the Lord want to help me? I need to get myself out of it. I'm not worthy of his help. I'm not worthy of a breakthrough. I've felt all that. Notice that the key word in all of that is "I."

I tend to put myself above the truth. To not hear the truth if it takes the word "I" out of the equation. I ask myself if I'm willing to be less selfish. Am I willing to say I'm sorry for wanting it my way? I ask the Lord to help me lose the weight, then wake up the next day discouraged. Then it becomes a me-thing again.

God could totally heal me of my weight problem. He could sweep in and make the weight disappear, but then what have I learned? Will I just put it all back on? Instead, I need to lay the selfishness aside. Just say, "Lord, I surrender."

I once read a letter to the newspaper. A woman wrote about her mom's death from obesity. She wondered why her mom did not love her enough to lose the weight, why she chose food over her own kids. If I want to be real with myself, then I have to see that overeating is selfish. It's something God and I need to work out. I need to realize life is about more than just me. I need to surrender.

Father, I want to surrender it all to you. Take my eyes off myself and help me to put them on you. Forgive me for my selfishness and greed. Make me willing to surrender to you now. In Jesus' name, amen.

by Nancy

March 4

Every way of a man is right in his own eyes, but the Lord weighs the heart.
Proverbs 21:2 ESV

Do not merely listen to the word, and so deceive yourselves. Do what it says.
James 1:22

There's a scene in the movie *What Women Want* where the Mel Gibson character is missing his new love interest (played by Helen Hunt) and he wanders around his apartment like he's lost. He stops and opens the fridge, stares at what's inside, and says something like, "What am I doing? She's not in there."

That scene describes perfectly what I'm going through when I want food that I don't need. What I really want, what I really *need* is never in the refrigerator unless I'm truly, physically hungry.

It took me a while to understand that wanting to eat more than I need is part of a *compulsion* to overeat. The compulsion comes from spiritual and emotional deficiencies that I'm trying to fill with food when I need to fill them with God. It's the same compulsion alcoholics have when they want to drink. My drug of choice just happens to be food.

I think I knew this at some level for a very long time. But knowing I had a problem is not the same as doing something about it. In other words, self-knowledge is not enough.

Father, I'm in trouble with food. I recognize it. I know I should eat healthy, and most of the time I even know what kinds of foods I should eat. But even that isn't enough to overcome my compulsions. Help me to turn my will and life over to you, including the food, so that I can take the actions you want me to take. The actions that are your will for me. In Jesus' name, amen.

by Debbie

March 5

Do not be deceived: God is not mocked,
for whatever one sows, that will he also reap.
Galatians 6:7 ESV

I do not understand what I do. For what I want to do
I do not do, but what I hate I do.
Romans 7:15

Self-knowledge is not enough to overcome an addiction. You can know what causes you to do something and still not be able to stop doing it. Over the years, I have studied (and learned) some things about nutrition. I've tried all kinds of diets and programs, including Atkins (low carb), Weight Watchers (low calorie), Kaiser's Freedom from Fat (low fat), TOPS (accountability), and others that were quite expensive, such as Jenny Craig and Nutrisystem.

They all worked in the short term. I lost some weight, but at most about fifteen pounds. Then once I (inevitably) grew tired of each program, I went back to eating the way I always had and gained the weight back. And over the years I gained and gained and gained until I was more than a hundred pounds overweight. At some level, I also understood that I had an addiction. I understood that somehow my overeating was linked to my emotions. I knew that it was compulsive. And yet just knowing that was not enough!

It took surrendering to God and a plan of action to finally come to terms with and overcome the compulsion. Even now I'm overcoming it day by day and doing it imperfectly. But I am overcoming. I do have victory, one day at a time.

Father, thank you for showing me another way. Help me to continue to surrender to you anew each day. In Jesus' name, amen.

by Debbie

March 6

And we know that in all things God works for the good of those who love him, who have been called according to his purpose.
Romans 8:28

Control can be an ugly word. Sometimes I wonder if I'm wearing myself out with controlling everything else in my life because of my lack of control with my eating. Maybe I don't want to deal with myself, and that makes me want to control everything else. But truthfully, most of it is not mine to control.

I have sometimes worn myself and my family out trying to make sure the house is perfect. My family has to be "just right," or I feel I've lost something along the way. My marriage has to be a shining example, or what good is it?

What would happen if my house wasn't so perfect? What would happen if my kids made mistakes just because they're human, and it really was no reflection on me? What would happen if I took the pressure off my husband and allowed him to just "be"? Would the world keep spinning?

My eyes should be on myself. I must be willing to see the plank in my own eye rather than the speck in yours. True freedom won't come by controlling everything else. It won't come by having to be the "strong" one. It comes only by believing God enough to let him bring us out of the prison of self.

The saddest thing about trying to control everything and everyone is that eventually it will all crash around us, because it's not ours to control.

Father, when I feel the urge to control everything, help me to turn it over to you instead. Help me to remember that only you are sovereign. Help me to surrender it all to you. In Jesus' name, amen.

by Nancy

March 7

For we are God's handiwork, created in Christ Jesus to do good works, which God prepared in advance for us to do.
Ephesians 2:10

The irony of seeking to discover my personal purpose in life is that it means that I must stop focusing on myself to do it. Self-centeredness has been a prime feature of my being, and it has manifested in a strong desire to control my own life. Like I've heard others say, I need to remind myself: "How's that workin' out for ya?" The idea is to become less self-centered and more God-centered. Do I really mean it when I say I've turned my will and my life over to God? Do I mean it when I say that God can do with me what he wills? What is it that I haven't yet surrendered to him? For much of my life the answer to that question was the food. I wanted to eat what I wanted, when I wanted, and how much.

In thinking about my purpose in life, I believe that we all have several. First, we are here on earth to learn. God has things he wants us to know. Second, we're meant to participate in his redemptive plan for us and for humanity. Third, we're meant to help our fellow human beings along the way and to allow some of them to help us. Fourth, we're meant to have fellowship with God, who wants to be our friend. Letting food be a substitute for a relationship with God means that I can't really be friends with him. I must turn it over. I must surrender.

Father, today I ask that you would help me to live out your purposes for my life. And thank you that every day, if I turn toward you and turn my life over to you, you'll continue to make me a better human being. In Jesus' name, amen.

by Debbie

March 8

Father, if you are willing, take this cup from me;
yet not my will, but yours be done.
Luke 22:42

I desire to do your will, my God; your law is within my heart.
Psalm 40:8

When I watch a movie like *Tortured for Christ*, I wonder how I would react if put in that person's place. My American life has been so comfortable by comparison. Would I be able to pray for my tormentors as Richard Wurmbrand did? Would I keep my faith? Doing so would mean doing God's will completely.

Yet for most of my life I've been full of self-will. And that's how I've lived it. Especially when it came to what I put in my mouth. Even now, I struggle with it. Each day I struggle with the willingness to surrender what I eat to God.

For someone like me, who started with more than a hundred pounds to lose, I've had no choice but to surrender. Without asking God what I should eat and what I should not, nothing would have changed. When I listen and do what God shows me, I do well. When I decide that I want to eat what I want when I want it, I fail utterly. When I first started, the idea of letting God choose my foods was a completely foreign concept. But once I started to let him guide me, I also started to have success. It's when I stomp my foot like a two-year-old and yell "mine" over some food or other that I again have difficulty.

Father, for much of my life I've been a two-year-old stomping my foot, whining for a yummy treat. But those treats have poisoned my body. Thank you for showing me a better way, for showing me how to surrender. Amen.

by Debbie

March 9

For I know that good itself does not dwell in me, that is,
in my sinful nature. For I have the desire to do what is good,
but I cannot carry it out. What a wretched man I am!
Who will rescue me from this body that is subject to death?
Thanks be to God, who delivers me through Jesus Christ our Lord!
Romans 7:18, 24–25

I like to read Christian romance novels. I finished one called *Beyond the Shadows* that really got me thinking. It's about a young widow who gets married again—to a man she discovers is an alcoholic. What really got me was the thoughts of the people who knew the couple. They saw what was happening but either ignored it or felt it was not their place to say anything.

In the novel, one of their friends had thoughts that I felt pertained to me with my overeating: "It's painful to watch the suffering of a beloved friend. She reminds me of a rubber ball, bouncing high, falling low, bouncing back again. One day faith-filled, hopeful, praying for all she was worth. The next she was in despair, looking to God, yet not expecting his answers, not even wanting to pray for her husband because of her anger. She chose to surrender with one hand and sought to control with the other."

That reminds me so much of myself with my struggle to stop overeating. I'm like a rubber ball. I do really well one day and the next I mess up big time. I get angry at myself, so I feel I cannot pray. And I don't want to pray about it. I surrender on one hand and want to keep control with the other. Lord, help me.

Father, please give me strength. Restore me to a new way of thinking and living. Give me wisdom. Help me when I can't help myself. In Jesus' name, amen.

by Nancy

March 10

"I have the right to do anything," you say—but not everything is beneficial. "I have the right to do anything"—but I will not be mastered by anything.
1 Corinthians 6:12

Not only so, but we also glory in our sufferings, because we know that suffering produces perseverance; perseverance, character; and character, hope.
Romans 5:3–4

When I'm craving a food that I know is a problem for me, it helps to do a contrary action. But I also need to deal with the feelings that are causing me to have those phantom hunger pains. I can get up and take a walk, have a diet soda or a cup of tea, brush my teeth, send a buddy a chatty e-mail, and—best of all—I can pray.

That's how I deal with this addiction. If I don't meet life as it comes, and things get buried, the feelings come out in the form of addictive behavior. Of that I'm certain. I have found that the number one feeling I ate over is frustration. I also ate over out-and-out anger, and sometimes out of resentment. Sometimes out of boredom, and sometimes because I was not enjoying what I was doing at work at the moment. Often, I was unhappy about something small. All were negative feelings that I couldn't or wouldn't deal with. Things I didn't want to feel.

It's worthwhile to look at this part of our lives and acknowledge it. And to know we're not alone. (I sometimes wonder if there's anybody in the entire world who's not addicted to something or other.) What I have learned is that my addiction ensures that I must drop to my knees and ask God to help me. Every time it rears its ugly head.

Father, thank you that addiction has forced me to rely on you. Amen.

by Debbie

March 11

"Why do you call me, 'Lord, Lord,' and do not do what I say?"
Luke 6:46

There's a wise (and truly funny) saying that I've often contemplated: *If I disagree with God, guess who's wrong?*

Have you ever argued with God? I have. Sometimes it's about something he doesn't want me to do. Sometimes it's about something he wants me to do. For example: He wants me to eat a healthy breakfast, something with fiber in it, like oatmeal. I'm not a big fan of oatmeal, so I tried to make a deal with God: I'll eat it four days a week. Do I always eat it all four of those days? No. Yet God is such a gentleman that he still allows me to make my own choice, even when my choice isn't good for me.

He often did this with his people. In the time of the Old Testament judges, God himself was Israel's king. Then the people asked God to give them a king so they'd be like the neighboring kingdoms. (That sounds familiar, doing something just to fit in.) God warned them having a king wouldn't be good for them, but they persisted, and he gave them what they wanted. And they experienced all the consequences God warned them about.

How many times have I given in to what I wanted rather than what God wanted for me? With food, there have been too many times to count. Yet there have been times when I *have* surrendered my will to God. When I *have* obeyed him rather than my own selfish desires. And whenever I have done that, he has blessed me.

So the next time I feel like arguing with God, I'll remember that phrase: *If I disagree with God, guess who's wrong?*

Father, today I surrender. Help me do your will, not my own. In Jesus' name, amen.

by Debbie

March 12

And just before the ev'ning in the cool of the day, They hear the voice of God as He is walking, And they can't abide His presence, so they try to hide away; But still they hear the sound as He is calling: "Adam, Adam, where are you?" In the stifling heat of summer now the gard'ner and his wife are in the field, And it seems that thorns and thistles are the only crop his struggles ever yield, He eats his meals in sorrow till he sinks into the dust whence he came, But all down through the ages he can hear his Maker calling out his name: "Adam, Adam, where are you?"

One of the songs I love to listen to is "Adam, Where Are You?" by Don Francisco. As I was listening, I thought, *My life is just like Adam's. Especially with the overeating.*

Adam and Eve knew they had done wrong. They hid from God. They knew they were naked and ashamed. Am I doing that? Am I hiding "behind the bush" of fat? I know what I do is wrong. I know that I need to change. Yet I hide, thinking deep within: *Please, Lord, don't find all that's buried beneath the fat.*

And yet he is still calling, "Beloved child, where are you?"

It starts out with a wonderful feeling. It feels so good to take that bite of candy. To drink that calorie-laden soda. How many times a day do I bow down at Satan's hand—because it feels good? And yet God is calling out, "Where are you?"

Thorns and thistles are all that we get in return. So many thorns. So much sadness. So much shame. Still prisoners to our own destruction. God is crying out, "Come in from the darkness before it's time to close the door. Where are you?"

Father, help me in my weakness and rebellion. Help me to want your way instead of mine. Help me to surrender to your perfect will for my life. In Jesus' name, amen.

by Nancy

March 13

Let us rejoice and be glad and give him glory! For the wedding of the Lamb has come, and his bride has made herself ready.
Revelation 19:7

I am my beloved's and my beloved is mine.
Song of Solomon 6:3

What does it mean to be a bride? A bride longs to marry and live with her groom. She aches to be with him. She is lonely without him. That makes me think of the empty place that's inside all of us. Addicts are always trying to fill that empty place with something other than what was meant to fill it.

For people who have a weight problem, that problem isn't actually the food they eat. The problem is that they're trying to fill an empty place within—with the wrong thing. The hunger they think they feel is a manifestation of that empty place inside.

Yet instead of filling it with God's presence and love, which is the only thing that can truly fill it up, we try to fill it by filling our stomachs, by enjoying the pleasures of certain tastes, salty and sweet, and textures, smooth and crunchy. And more. Always more, because it's never enough.

It works for a time—all substances do. Alcohol does. Marijuana does. Heroin does. Food does. Until it doesn't work anymore. Until it becomes harmful rather than helpful.

There is an empty place inside that only God can fill. If you fill it with the right thing, you won't need to try to fill it with something else that will never fully satisfy. Only the presence of the Groom satisfies the bride.

Lord, help me to always remember that you are my only beloved. Amen.

by Debbie

March 14

I am the true vine, and my Father is the gardener. He cuts off every branch in me that bears no fruit, while every branch that does bear fruit he prunes so that it will be even more fruitful.
John 15:1–2

When I started this weight-loss journey, I was going to conquer the fat. I was taking on the world! I knew I was going to make it because I WANTED IT! And you know what? People were amazed because I said how fun it was. I loved every minute. I enjoyed not pigging out; I enjoyed not feeling full all the time; I enjoyed knowing that I was being obedient to the Lord; I enjoyed picturing myself thin and running and playing.

Then suddenly I wavered, and things got harder. Satan likes to spread discouragement. I started thinking, *You've been at this a year now and you've only lost thirty-six pounds.* That led to another thought: *You aren't going to make it in this lifetime.*

In the end, victory is not about me and my willpower. It's about being willing to trust in God and *his* power. God knows what he's doing. I will trust him!

Today I'm going to search my heart and see what's there that could be hindering me. Am I scared to lose weight for fear that people will treat me differently? Is the weight a way of avoiding things in my life? Am I covering up my past in the fat? Tough questions, for which I don't always have answers. I do know that God wants ALL of this weight-loss journey, not just the parts I want to give him. He doesn't need my fragments. He wants ALL of me.

Father, help me to be willing to give you all of me so that I can have victory in your power, not my own. In Jesus' name, amen.

by Nancy

March 15

Yes, my soul, find rest in God; my hope comes from him. Trust in him at all times, you people; pour out your hearts to him, for God is our refuge.
Psalm 62:5,8

And the peace of God, which transcends all understanding, will guard your hearts and your minds in Christ Jesus.
Philippians 4:7

I had a revelation, something I already knew, but hadn't practiced regularly: I can be free from worry and self-pity if I truly trust the Lord. If I say, "Okay, God, whatever happens, I know that it will be okay, because it's all in your plan, and because you love me." That is such a freeing statement. If I truly take it to heart, I know there is no reason to worry anymore, because God is there to take care of me. Not that I can do that perfectly, but it does help to at least let some of the things go that I'm worrying about. But I must be willing to say to God, "Whatever you want, I'll accept." It seems like a tall order, but ultimately it sets me free.

I have also meditated on the serenity prayer: God, grant me the serenity to accept the things I cannot change, the courage to change the things I can, and the wisdom to know the difference. It's simple, but profound, and if I truly pray it and mean it, it works. If I can get my needs met by God through prayer and meditation, and he really will meet me when I reach out to him, then I won't need the candy and Little Debbies and sweetened cereal. He will be enough.

Father, help me to trust you completely, help me to turn my life over to you. When I do that, I know that I no longer need to worry, and I can live with a heart full of peace. In Jesus' name, amen.

by Debbie

March 16

Praise be to the God and Father of our Lord Jesus Christ, the Father of compassion and the God of all comfort, who comforts us in all our troubles.
2 Corinthians 1:3–4

I have often wondered why we overeat. I really think part of my problem is that in some way I feel this is an area that I have complete say. Nobody can tell me what to do. If I want to eat, I will eat.

Sometimes I feel pushed in every direction. I have to have the mommy face on, then I have to have the wife face on, then I have to have the church face on, then I have to have the women's ministry face on. Not that I'm different in each of them. But in all those things I'm not in control. My mommy face is controlled by the kids or grandkids. My wife face is controlled by my husband. And so on.

The eating seems to be the one thing that's mine. Can you tell I was raised in the seventies? The ME generation. Yet I really think it's time to get rid of that selfishness, because I really am not doing ME any good. I'm only hurting ME!

I actually love being a mommy. I love being involved in church. I love being a wife. But can I love being me?

A friend wrote to me once, saying she thinks sometimes we find comfort in our eating, and even in our extra weight. It has been with us so long, and the food has been a comfort for so long that once we finally stop, we're putting it to death. And our response is often: *Oh no! What will comfort me now?* We all know the answer. It's time to let God do the comforting. He wants to do that for us. We need to quit giving that job to food.

Father, help me to turn to you for my comfort—not to food. In Jesus' name, amen.

by Nancy

March 17

There is a time for everything, and a season for every activity under the heavens: a time to be silent and a time to speak. . . . everything God does will endure forever; nothing can be added to it and nothing taken from it.
Ecclesiastes 3:1,7,14

Sometimes the best thing, the wisest thing to do is nothing. That is usually the case when I want to say something (or on social media, write something) when it would be better not to respond at all. But there are other times when it's vital to take action. If I'm craving food when I should be done eating for the day, for example, what am I really hungry for? My go-to anytime I'm feeling empty, and sometimes just because I'm feeling *something*, is to reach for something to eat.

It's been my way of comforting myself for a very long time. Maybe I learned it as a child. Maybe even as a baby. Maybe not until I was a teenager. When it happened, or even how, doesn't matter as much as what I choose to do about it now.

When I read *The Purpose-Driven Life* I learned, "It's not about me." If I want to discover my purpose in life, I need to remember that it starts with my Creator. I believed that for a long time, but I never really lived it. I finally realized that isn't it about time I did? The irony of discovering my personal purpose in life, which I actually have longed for, is that it means that I must stop focusing on myself to do it. Instead, I must focus on God and what he wants me to do. I must focus on his will for my life.

And why shouldn't I? After all, he knows everything, including what's best for me.

Father, teach me the right time to do everything, including when to speak and when to be quiet. Teach me your ways and help me follow them. Amen.

by Debbie

March 18

Cast your cares on the Lord and he will sustain you;
he will never let the righteous be shaken.
Psalm 55:22

Now to him who is able to do immeasurably more than all we ask or imagine, according to his power that is at work within us, to him be glory in the church and in Christ Jesus throughout all generations, for ever and ever! Amen.
Ephesians 3:20

Am I controlling the food? Or is food controlling me? Control can be such an ugly word. In my own life, there have been times when I've had to have complete control. Control over my marriage. Over my kids. And, yes, even control over God (as if that's possible).

Yet, ironically, I also feel sometimes that life is completely out of control. I try hard to keep it all under my thumb, but that causes me to get so worn out. It makes me feel weary all the time. So maybe, just maybe, it's time to relinquish control.

If I give over control to the Father, just maybe things will fall into place in my life. With my marriage and children. In my life with the Lord. And with the weight-loss journey.

Just maybe God has a better plan for how the extra weight will come off than I could ever imagine. Maybe I should give him a chance to prove that he is perfectly able to work abundantly within my life. Control really is not as glamorous as Satan would have us believe. Let's give that control to the Lord and let's be set free once and for all!

Father, help me to always remember that being in control is an illusion and that you are sovereign over everything. In Jesus' name, amen.

by Nancy

March 19

But seek first the kingdom of God and his righteousness, and all these things will be added to you. Therefore, do not be anxious about tomorrow, for tomorrow will be anxious for itself. Sufficient for the day is its own trouble.
Matthew 6:33–34 ESV

What areas of my life am I holding back from God? Food, time, money, social media? I have almost always held things back due to fear. Fear of losing control. Fear of being lonely. Fear of not having enough money to meet my needs. Fear of losing someone. Fear of illness or death. But what is F.E.A.R.? False Expectations Appearing Real.

Perhaps that's why God tells us so many times throughout the Bible to "Fear not." Every day I have a choice about whether to continue to live in fear or to begin to live in trust. And trusting in God almost always means giving up control.

In *The Purpose Driven Life* we read, "Surrendering is not for cowards or doormats . . . it doesn't mean giving up rational thinking. . . . Instead of trying harder, you trust more. . . . There is a moment of surrender, and there is the practice of surrender. The problem with a living sacrifice is that it can crawl off the altar, so you have to resurrender your life fifty times a day."

And C. S. Lewis wrote, "The more we let God take us over, the more truly ourselves we become—because he made us." That means that I don't have to fear giving up control to God. I can trust him with everything that I have and everything that I am.

Father, build my trust in you so that I no longer have to fear. Thank you for meeting my needs so that I can learn to trust you more. And when I inevitably run into life's troubles, help me to continue to trust you, no matter what. In Jesus' name, amen.

by Debbie

March 20

All those gathered here will know that it is not by the sword or the spear that the Lord saves; for the battle is the Lord's.
1 Samuel 17:47

God tells us to cast ALL our cares on Him. Nowhere in my Bible does it say to cast half or three-quarters of them. Yet sometimes I'm quick to say, "Okay, Lord, please take this" and then twenty minutes later I start worrying about it again.

God showed me that is exactly what I have done with this weight-loss journey. I tried to do it on my own. Many times I prayed in the morning and by noon I had already taken it back. In reality, he wants us to follow his leading and not try to figure it all out on our own.

In 1 Samuel it's clear that the battle is the Lord's. Once we repent and take the action of true repentance, then the battle becomes the Lord's. Do you think Satan is going to roll over and say, "I give up"? No. He's going to fight all the harder. But we can't go against the adversary except with God.

On our own we may practically starve ourselves in our attempt to lose weight. We may think we should exercise three hours a day. But the battle is the Lord's, and we need to follow what he wants us to do. When you first decide to do this, you might feel like I did at first, like a scared child who grab's Daddy's hand and hides behind Mommy's skirts. Instead, let Daddy fight the battle for you. The battle is the Lord's!

Lord, thank you that you are a big Daddy God who will go before me to fight a battle that I can't really even see. Food is sometimes my Goliath, and I'm just a little David with a sling. But it wasn't David who won that battle, it was you, giving him success. Please help me in the same way. In Jesus' name, amen.

by Nancy

March 21

If any of you lacks wisdom, you should ask God, who gives generously to all without finding fault, and it will be given to you.
James 1:5

When I was attending graduate school, we went through an exercise that helped us define our two most important personal values. Mine are faith and wisdom. I was reminded about wisdom again when reading a scripture devotional that I received as a high school graduation present from the pastor of my church (many, many years ago now).

The scriptures listed on my birthday talk about taking a stance, living whole-heartedly for Jesus, and putting away the things of the world to follow him: *Dear children, keep away from anything that might take God's place in your hearts. 1 John 5:21, TLB.*

In order to do that, I must seek wisdom. I have prayed and asked God, "Please give me wisdom," as I have much desired both wisdom and discernment. Why? Because I've lacked both for a good portion of my life.

Most of my life, I have wanted to live my way. And when I did that, things usually didn't turn out well—either for me or for those around me. For me, wisdom has meant giving in to God. Turning my life over to him. Learning to eat the way he wants me to eat. That's because when I'm in control, I'm sure to mess it up. And I have messed it up. Turning it over means praying each morning for God to give me wisdom and direction. It means saying thy will, not mine be done.

Jesus, I need to make you Lord of my life. Not just once, but I need to do it again every morning. Please help to me to do your will always. Amen.

by Debbie

March 22

Their destiny is destruction, their god is their stomach, and their glory is in their shame. Their mind is set on earthly things. But our citizenship is in heaven. And we eagerly await a Savior from there, the Lord Jesus Christ, who, by the power that enables him to bring everything under his control, will transform our lowly bodies so that they will be like his glorious body.
Philippians 3:19–21

That says it all doesn't it? Their god is their stomach, and their destiny is destruction. Wow! What do you want your destiny to be? Early death? High cholesterol? Diabetes?

Or would you like a long life, good times with your family, a healthy level of self-esteem?

God says here that to transform our bodies we have to bring everything under his control. Are we willing to give up that control? Are we willing to allow him to transform our bodies and make them just like his?

I say, "Yes, Lord! Transform me!"

I must make God my Father, my only true God. I must let my stomach know that it will no longer rule me. What's a little bit of growling? I can bring it under his control. What's a little bit of discomfort? I can bring it under his control.

Even though St. Paul is talking about the future—about our future bodies after the resurrection of the saints at the end of the age—I'm okay with thinking about now too. If I give God the control, just maybe I can have a small taste of what it's like to have the glorious body he has promised!

Father, if I call you Lord, then help me to make you Lord of everything in my life. Lord, I keep saying the same words over and over again: Help me! Help me to want to be obedient, even when it's not easy. In Jesus' name, amen.

by Nancy

March 23

During the days of Jesus' life on earth, he offered up prayers and petitions with fervent cries and tears to the one who could save him from death, and he was heard because of his reverent submission. Son though he was, he learned obedience from what he suffered and, once made perfect, he became the source of eternal salvation for all who obey.
Hebrews 5:7–10

We are to follow Christ's example. What did he do? He prayed, he suffered, and he was obedient. He did those things because he was perfect, but it goes further than that. He did those things because he loved God, and God loved him (one of the mysteries of the Trinity).

What does that mean for me? It means that I become willing to pray, to be obedient, and, yes, sometimes even to suffer (like giving up some of my favorite foods?), because I love God. Yet I can only love God, because he first loved me. It's Jesus' love that compels me, and his love in me that enables me. I am the weakest of the weak, and it's only through God's help that I can do what he asks.

Now that I have Christ living in me, if I step into sin again, it's usually because either I'm weak or because I want to. In other words, either I just don't have the strength on my own, or my heart is rebellious and I want to do what I want rather than what God knows is best for me.

It's laughable that sometimes I think I know better than God, but sometimes I still do. It's only when I surrender fully that thing I'm holding onto so tightly that I can finally have any success at all.

Lord, make me willing to surrender my life fully to you. Amen.

by Debbie

March 24

But seek first his kingdom and his righteousness,
and all these things will be given to you as well.
Matthew 6:33

This morning I pictured a plate of food. On it were meat, potatoes, and some vegetables. As you would normally see on someone's plate in the Midwest where I live, the meat was the biggest item. Then the potatoes. Then the vegetables.

Then I realized that each of them is healthy. Each one has a place in my life. But one was bigger than the rest. I then thought, *What is the "meat" in my life? How do I choose my priorities?*

We know the "meat" should be God. The "potatoes" should be our family. The "vegetables" are everything else. But is that how it truly is? Have our diets taken over so that they're more important than our family?

A diet can take over so much of my life. I know when I step on the scale, and I have gained, I can be irritable for the rest of the day. If I had a bad day at my job, maybe my family paid the price when I got home. I don't always treat people with the grace they deserve.

We shouldn't put anything ahead of God. Not our food, not even our diet. Will I keep begging him for answers, yet when his still small voice is leading me, am I just too stubborn to hear him? Or am I too rebellious to follow him?

Today it's time for me to look at my plate and make sure I have prioritized it the way *he* wants. God should be my meat every day. My family should be a priority. And then all the other things in my life will fall into place.

Father, teach me to make you the most important thing always. Amen.

by Nancy

March 25

The Lord had said to Abram, "Go from your country, your people and your father's household to the land I will show you. After this, the word of the Lord came to Abram in a vision: "Do not be afraid, Abram. I am your shield, your very great reward."
Genesis 12:1, 15:1

My pastor once taught, "God has called us to faithfulness, not to outcomes. The perpetual lie of the enemy is that we can do this on our own power. God told Abram, 'I need you to step out in faith before you can see that anything has happened.' It means faithfully showing up day after day and doing what God shows me to do. It means doing the little things that God has called you to do today."

That made me think about what God might be calling me to do in obedience to him. Has he called me to eat oatmeal for breakfast (so I'll have more fiber in my diet)? Has he called me to stop eating sugar? Has he called me to give up foods that will increase my appetite later?

Abram took steps in faith. He went to Canaan. He believed God's promise that his descendants would become a great nation even though his wife was childless. God has promised that he'll give us success IF we obey him. That includes success in overcoming compulsive eating and in attaining a healthy body weight. What has God asked you to do? And what has God promised you?

Father, help me to walk in obedience to you, even when I don't know why you have asked me to do something. Thank you for your promises. Thank you for promising me success—if I'm willing to obey. In Jesus' name, amen.

by Debbie

March 26

What shall we say, then? Shall we go on sinning so that grace may increase? By no means! We are those who have died to sin; how can we live in it any longer? For we know that our old self was crucified with him so that the body ruled by sin might be done away with, that we should no longer be slaves to sin—because anyone who has died has been set free from sin. In the same way, count yourselves dead to sin but alive to God in Christ Jesus. Therefore, do not let sin reign in your mortal body so that you obey its evil desires. Do not offer any part of yourself to sin as an instrument of wickedness, but rather offer yourselves to God as those who have been brought from death to life; and offer every part of yourself to him as an instrument of righteousness. For sin shall no longer be your master, because you are not under the law, but under grace.
Romans 6:1–2, 11–14

If only I could see that sin leads only to death. I have let sin tell me what to do my whole life. If only I could teach myself that it is a dead language. That sin will always hold me in bondage.

There is only one way I can break free. It will never let me go, not until the Lord breaks the chains. It's time to let God tell me what to do. Then I can truly walk in the freedom that he has for me. Then I can walk without the chains of fat, without the lack of energy and all the other problems that come with obesity.

I really am feeling the pricking from the Lord. I'm hearing that still, small voice encouraging me. Will I listen?

Father, thank you for helping me to understand the depravity of my own sin. Thank you that knowing the truth has led me to want to walk in obedience to you and your word. Guide me, direct me, show me what you want me to do now. Show me how to live in your grace, your mercy, and your strength. Help me all along the way. In Jesus' name, amen.

by Nancy

March 27

So he did what the Lord had told him.
1 Kings 17:5

I have recently been studying the prophet Elijah. One thing that stood out to me about him is his audacity. He had the audacity to obey God even when what God was asking him to do seemed strange or counterintuitive.

I want to be like Elijah. When God asks me to do something, I want to be willing to do it. One thing I did that I never thought I could do was to give up refined sugar. It's been two years now, and I have no regrets. It was one of my best life decisions. The health benefits have been immense, and I now see the profound wisdom of it.

To do it, I had to be willing to obey God rather than stubbornly stick to what I wanted. But the way Elijah was different than I have been, was that he was willing to obey each directive from God, all the time. In 1 Kings 17 and 18, each time "the word of the Lord" came to Elijah telling him to do something, he immediately went and did it. No questions asked. Up till now, I've been more like Jonah. When God asked Jonah to preach to Nineveh, he ran away. Which is how he ended up in the belly of a giant fish. I've done that far too many times.

I'm sure God has more things he wants to refine in my diet. Will I be willing to do them when he asks? I pray so. The Lord can help me obey when I should, if I ask. If.

Father, help me to be obedient, even when I'm reluctant. Remind me that you are far wiser than I am and that, to you, obedience is the one true way I can show you that I love you. Remind me to ask you for help, always. In Jesus' name, amen.

by Debbie

March 28

The Israelites said to them, "If only we had died by the Lord's hand in Egypt! There we sat around pots of meat and ate all the food we wanted, but you have brought us out into this desert to starve this entire assembly to death."
Then the Lord said to Moses, "I will rain down bread from heaven for you. The people are to go out each day and gather enough for that day.
Exodus 16:3–4

The very next words after that passage struck me as I read them: *In this way I will test them and see whether they will follow my instructions.* What I noticed specifically was that the Israelites wondered why they couldn't have died in the COMFORT of their food. They too related food to their comfort. And they were willing to die for it. Am I willing to die for the comfort of food? If I'm being completely honest, I would have to say yes, I am. I know exactly what this extra weight is doing to my body, yet I stubbornly keep on eating. Shoving that food in, bite by bite.

The scripture then talks about how God chose to test the people to see if they would do what is right. That made me wonder if he tests me. I think he does, daily.

I once wrote a prayer out in my food journal telling the Lord what I would work on that day. I told him what I needed his help with. Then within a few hours, that was shot. Maybe he wanted to see how serious I was about doing the right thing. I failed. But that doesn't mean I'll fail tomorrow. I'll get right back at it. I won't give up, because I know he hasn't given up on me.

Father, I know one of the reasons you test me is to remind me that only you can overcome sin. Only you have the power to show me what needs to change and to change it. Help me remember that only by surrendering to you can I overcome anything. In Jesus' name, amen.

by Nancy

March 29

You were taught, with regard to your former way of life, to put off your old self, which is being corrupted by its deceitful desires; to be made new in the attitude of your minds; and to put on the new self, created to be like God in true righteousness and holiness.
Ephesians 4:22–24

Since this Bible verse reminds me of repentance, I looked up the definition of "repent" on merriam-webster.com: 1: to turn from sin and dedicate oneself to the amendment of one's life; 2a: to feel regret or contrition; b: to change one's mind. Interestingly, repent can also be used as an adjective, as in a *repent vine*. As in to lie flat on the ground, to be *prostrate*. That's a lot to think about.

What I also noticed about this verse is that it doesn't say that God is the one who takes our old self from us and clothes us with a new self (although I think he can and does do that). But it asks *us* to do an action—to put something off and to put something else on. Even though I'm powerless over what some foods do to me, I still have some responsibility to take certain actions to overcome my addiction and my compulsive eating.

I have a responsibility to make a decision to turn my will and my life over to God. To ask God what his will is for my life. To ask God to renew my mind. And then I have a responsibility to obey. That's the part where I put on the new self—through obedience to God's will. That may mean giving up some of my favorite foods. It may mean weighing and measuring what I eat. It may mean listening to the wisdom of others who have lost weight and kept it off and following their advice.

Father, show me your will regarding my food choices, and then give me the strength to do what you have asked. In Jesus' name, amen.

by Debbie

March 30

The mind governed by the flesh is hostile to God; it does not submit to God's law, nor can it do so. Those who are in the realm of the flesh cannot please God. You, however, are not in the realm of the flesh but are in the realm of the Spirit, if indeed the Spirit of God lives in you.
Romans 8:7,9

In the Christian romance novel *Beyond the Shadows*, a man, an ex-addict, came to the rescue of the heroine's husband, an alcoholic. The husband talks about what happened: "No one sets out to be an alcoholic. The next thing I knew, I didn't need stress or a problem for a reason to drink. I'd gulp down a drink or two. Maybe three. But I could handle three. I never felt a buzz. Never did anything stupid. I could still control when I started drinking. Or so I thought. Denial with a capital D."

How many times do we really need an excuse to eat? I want to blame it on *something*, but do I really eat extra food only when I'm stressed? Only when I have a problem? If I'm honest, I have to say no. I don't need an excuse. How many times have I eaten when people were not around—so that I could have more when they're there, and they won't know that I had extra already?

In the novel, the husband's friend says, "Sobriety is the first step. We've got to believe God can restore us to a better way of living and thinking. We ask him to give us the strength to change. We ask him for the wisdom to know how and what to change."

God, I offer myself to you, to build with me and to do with me as you will. Relieve me of the bondage of self, that I may better do your will. Take away my difficulties, that victory over them may bear witness to those I would help of your power, your love, and your way of life. Amen. (AA's Third Step Prayer)

by Nancy

March 31

Then Jesus told his disciples, "If anyone would come after me, let him deny himself and take up his cross and follow me."
Matthew 16:24 ESV

Surrender. In our culture, that word brings up images of waving a white flag, an abject sense of defeat that comes from losing a war, or a sense of triumph as we watch an enemy surrender, knowing that we have won. But in God's kingdom it means something else entirely.

For me, surrender has been the recognition that I am human and that God is God. He is the Creator, and I am the created. He knows everything about me, and I don't really know myself at all. He knows what I need, while I only think I know what I need. What I think I need is usually what I *want* . . . and most of the time, reaching for what I want hasn't worked out so well for me.

This is true for me about the food I choose to eat. For most of my adult life, I've eaten what I wanted, when I wanted, as often as I wanted. The results of that willful self-indulgence have not been pretty: a bloated, grossly overweight, unhealthy body.

The first step toward surrender of my self-will was to recognize how wrong I was. I had to recognize that my choices, were destructive, and that if I kept going down the same path, I would get the same results. The second step was to recognize that God has the answers. The third step was to surrender my will and my life to God, including the food I choose to eat each day.

When I did those things, I was finally able to let go of the overeating and let go of a good portion of the extra weight.

Jesus, I surrender all. And tomorrow I'll have to do it again. Give me the strength to give up my self-will and surrender my life to you. Amen.

by Debbie

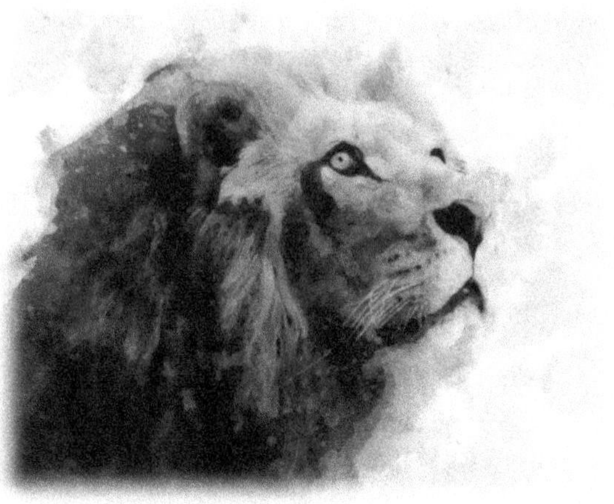

COURAGE

We must be fearless in
facing the truth about ourselves.

Cry of Our Hearts

April 1

Coveting, wickedness, deceit, sensuality, envy, slander, pride, foolishness.
All these evil things come from within, and they defile a person.
Mark 7:22–23 ESV

I acknowledged my sin to you, and I did not cover my iniquity;
I said, "I will confess my transgressions to the Lord,"
and you forgave the iniquity of my sin.
Psalm 32:5 ESV

Confessing sin to God and repenting of it is scriptural, but what I didn't realize was that holding onto unconfessed sin was holding me back from victory over compulsive overeating. I'd heard the saying, "You're only as sick as your secrets," but I didn't understand how true that is.

I also didn't understand myself very well. I knew that I couldn't actually keep anything secret from God, though I often acted like I could. But there were things I had done that I had forgotten. Sins and mistakes that I had never actively confessed to God or another human being. There were things I'd done that caused me to continually carry a burden of guilt and shame.

We all have those kinds of burdens, and we all need to be relieved of them. Anger and resentment, dishonesty, fear, false pride, self-centeredness, sexual sin—even negative thinking. It's important to confront it all. It takes courage to do that. And it has taken me more than one session of thinking and praying before I got all of it out. And because of the way the human heart is, I'm sure that more will be revealed that I'll have to confess. My advice? Make a list and confess it now. It will set you free.

Father, give me the courage to confess everything to you today. Amen.

by Debbie

April 2

He cuts off every branch in me that bears no fruit, while every branch that does bear fruit he prunes so that it will be even more fruitful.
John 15:2

I'd love to say we are purified through prosperity, but for better or worse we are purified through difficulty. He is . . . pruning away our rough edges so that we can be presented spotless and pure. As women know, physical beauty can be painful . . . our spiritual beauty is no different.
Hillary Morgan Ferrer

I don't know about how others have experienced overcoming compulsive overeating, but the most difficult part of the pruning process for me has been twofold: 1) surrendering my will about food to God, and 2) remembering to pray first before acting on a tempting thought about food. Yet I know these two actions work, because they work each time I do them.

My biggest problem is not lack of willpower. Quite the opposite. I have *too much* willpower. Another way of putting it is that I'm full of self-will. I want to eat like I always have and still lose weight. I want to blame everything else except my own actions for being overweight. I want to go through my day without having to pay attention to every little thing I eat. It's too much work to weigh and measure my food! It's too much work to change my habits! It's takes too much effort to write down every morsal that goes in my mouth. Who can live like that?!

But that's insane thinking. If I continue to do what I've always done, I'll continue to be like I've always been. It's only through having the courage to change that I will succeed.

Father, give me the courage and the willingness to change today. *Amen.*

by Debbie

April 3

God will take care of your tomorrow too. Live one day at a time.
Matthew 6:24 TLB

How many of you are commitment phobic? I know I am. If I think of something as a lifelong obligation, I run away—as fast as I can. The thought terrifies me that I may have to work at something for the rest of my life. My heart races, and I feel panic. I've heard that instead of dieting, we should make a lifestyle change. That does not give me a lot of hope that my "diet" will ever end. But there is hope; I can stop thinking of the word "change" and replace it with the idea of living in a healthier way.

I don't think God wants me to be bound by losing weight. That makes me think of a commercial I once saw that showed people dragging their bathroom scales behind them like a ball and chain. That's so *real*, isn't it? So many of us do that in one way or another. I have become shackled to "dieting." I've been shackled to "trying to become healthy."

I believe God has a much simpler plan. He says it right there in his word: "Don't worry about tomorrow." Whew! You mean I don't have to worry about what I'll weigh tomorrow?

We can all try something new today. We can just take today as today. Tomorrow will come eventually. But I don't have to be anxious for it. I can take today as it is and do my best. I can wake up in the morning and say, "This is the day the Lord has made!" I can choose to do what he wants me to do today.

Father, you can take away my anxiety and give me the courage to face each day as it comes. You can help me not to worry about tomorrow, because tomorrow will take care of itself. Give me your peace and your guidance each day. In Jesus' name, amen.

by Nancy

April 4

But as for you, be strong and do not give up,
for your work will be rewarded.
2 Chronicles 15:7

"Do not be afraid, you who are highly esteemed," he said. "Peace!
Be strong now; be strong." When he spoke to me, I was strengthened.
Daniel 10:19

It takes courage to face myself. It also takes courage to be willing to make a significant change in my life, like completely changing the way I eat. About two years ago, while going to a twelve-step program, I made the decision to give up refined sugar. I did it because I heard from people at meetings that it worked for them for long-term weight loss, and that's what I wanted. When I went into those meetings, what I really wanted was to lose weight. And I still do. But what has changed over time is that I also want to deal with what was causing me to overeat. And that takes courage too.

I deal with my compulsive eating by spending time working the twelve steps, which are based in Christian principles. One of the steps involves having the courage to face those things that have been causing me to stuff my feelings down with food. Once I asked, God brought things to mind that I needed to address. For me it's primarily been rebellion and self-will. Those "forces" are strong with me, and that hasn't been a good thing.

I don't always have courage, though, so I often have to ask for it. I frequently need to say the serenity prayer:

God, grant me the serenity to accept the things I cannot change, the courage to change the things I can, and the wisdom to know the difference. Amen.

by Debbie

April 5

When I am afraid, I put my trust in you.
Psalm 56:3

Peace I leave with you; my peace I give you. I do not give to you as the world gives. Do not let your hearts be troubled and do not be afraid.
John 14:27

The Lord said to me, "If you let fear creep into your heart, it will cause you to give up fighting for the best. Fear will cause you to settle. Fear will tell you that the price is too high, the road is too hard, the promise is too difficult to obtain." All we have to do is believe in him; he will do the rest.

Has fear caused you to settle? This can apply to so many areas of our lives. Finances, weight, marriage, children—the list could go on and on.

Let's face it—there are many fears in losing weight. Once we start the journey, life as we know it will not be the same. Things will change. We will change. And then there is the greatest fear: of not being successful at it.

So sometimes I think I'll just settle. I'll do the best I can, and when it seems I can't go any further, then I guess I'll just be happy the way things are. But that's WRONG! I shouldn't settle for anything less than full success.

God can show me my fears, and—more importantly—I can allow him to lead me through the healing and deliverance from those fears. I may not always believe it, but God says I'm worth it!

Father, your perfect love can drive out the fear in me. Give me courage in the face of my fears. May it be so! In Jesus' name, amen!

by Nancy

April 6

Anyone who listens to the word but does not do what it says is like someone who looks at his face in a mirror and, after looking at himself, goes away and immediately forgets what he looks like. But whoever looks intently into the perfect law that gives freedom and continues in it—not forgetting what they have heard, but doing it—they will be blessed in what they do.
James 1:23–25

Sometimes it's important to "act as if." At first I was really uncomfortable with all the changes I was making to my diet. It all felt so strange to me, like I was almost ready to do what I needed to do, but not quite. My eating wasn't the only habit I was changing. I was also weighing and measuring my food and using a food app to keep track of what I ate. I was going to meetings, making phone calls, writing in a journal, and reading literature that would help me in my weight-loss journey.

Along the way I was reminded of actor Michael Landon the last time he was on *The Tonight Show* just before he died of pancreatic cancer. He knew he was sick, and yet he was being positive—overly bright and sparkly—about it. He didn't last much longer after that.

That's how I felt at first. Like I was going through the motions, and it didn't feel right at all. It felt like I was living somebody else's life. But I continued to "act as if" it was my life until it actually felt like my life again. And I did get comfortable with it eventually. So will you.

Father, you gave us strong commandments about obeying you and your word. Put a new heart in me that wants to keep them. You want me to eat in a way that will allow me to attain a healthy body weight—so please also give me the courage to do the things I need to do to get there. In Jesus' name, amen.

by Debbie

April 7

So do not fear, for I am with you; do not be dismayed,
for I am your God. I will strengthen you and help you;
I will uphold you with my righteous right hand.
Isaiah 41:10

I was one of those people who thought that fear was a good thing. After all, doesn't the Bible say to fear God? In the Hebrew and Greek, the sense behind the word "fear" is that we are to reverence him. Honor him. Respect him. Stand in awe of him. That's one kind of fear.

But the Lord also says, "Don't be afraid!" Of what, then? Failure? Success? Economic insecurity? Illness? Death? There are so many things to be afraid of that I couldn't possibly list them all. The truth is—that kind of fear is bondage. It has a hold on us that we must allow God to deal with. Or we will be a slave to obesity the rest of our lives.

Isaiah tells us, "I will strengthen you and help you." Are we willing to allow God to help us? To strengthen us? Or do we want to continue to walk this path alone?

Growing up, I always felt that if I made a mistake it was up to me to fix it. I'm sure I said that to my children too. So onward I wandered, trying to fix things myself, but that often got me nowhere. The glorious thing about God is that he understands. He doesn't tell me how I screwed up and that I have make it better myself. Instead, he grabs my hand and says, "Walk with me. Allow me to guide you. Allow me to help you fix it."

Father, help me to remember to run to you today. When you reach out to me, let me see it so I can grab hold and take strength and courage from you as I walk with you hand in hand. In Jesus' name, amen.

by Nancy

April 8

For my iniquities have gone over my head;
like a heavy burden, they are too heavy for me.
Psalm 38:4 ESV

One of the things I have learned on this journey is that I must have the courage to deal with those parts of my life that I've been ignoring. When I first started, the Lord reminded me that I had done something I shouldn't and that if I didn't correct it, it was something that would keep me from succeeding in staying true to the eating plan he wanted me to pursue.

In other words, I was going to eat over it, much like an alcoholic might drink over something, because I hadn't dealt with it; I hadn't made things right. At first I resisted, but I did take care of it, and it freed me up to begin my plan successfully.

Another time, I had been eating the same way as usual, and yet just a little while after eating I felt empty, as if I were hungry again. But the Lord revealed to me that I wasn't physically hungry, I was emotionally and spiritually hungry, because I had been frustrated about several circumstances at home and at work.

So, I took action—I prayed and I talked to someone instead of eating—and somehow I felt full again. I wasn't hungry anymore. And yet I'm still sometimes tempted to add extra food to my meal or snack, because I worry about being hungry later. When that happens, I have to take an action again—something other than what I'm tempted to do at that moment.

Father, there are things that block my relationship with you. When they do, remind me to deal with them before they fester and get worse, just like a wound might if I don't clean it out and apply medicine so that it can heal. Please, Lord, give me courage to always face the truth and act on it. Amen.

by Debbie

April 9

In the multitude of my anxieties within me, Your comforts delight my soul.
Psalm 94:19

Fear not, for I have redeemed you; I have called you by name, you are mine.
Isaiah 43:1 ESV

Over and over again God has had to pound certain things into my head. It seems he does it through repetition.

Dealing with fear is one of those things. He once had me make a list of the fears in my life. As he brought each one to mind, it was an eye-opening experience. I sat and made the list, and it kept going and going. And going. I just did not realize all the different fears that have run rampant in my life.

Most of them stem from who I believe I am. What I erroneously think of myself has led to much havoc in my life. If I think badly of myself, then how can I have a good life? If I continually see myself as a failure, then I'll probably continue to fail. If I fear that I won't succeed at losing the weight, then I probably won't.

Yet I'm the daughter of the King. That makes me royalty. Now we should not run around with our noses up in the air, but we should be proud that Jesus is our King.

Do you see yourself as inadequate? As defeated? Afraid? The truth of who we are in Christ will indeed set us free. Read Chapters 1 and 2 of Ephesians; they tell you who you are in Christ. Study that and watch and wait and then be amazed at how differently you'll start seeing yourself and the truth of how your life actually is.

King Jesus, thank you for always working so hard to open my eyes to the truth of who I am in you. That gives me courage. Thank you, Amen.

by Nancy

April 10

As far as the east is from the west,
so far has he removed our transgressions from us.
Psalm 103:12

One of the things I have had to learn in this weight-loss journey is to forgive myself for the sins of the past. I've had to forgive myself for eating too much, for all my failures at all the diets I have ever tried, and even for weighing too much.

One way I've been able to do that is by recognizing what God's word says about my sins and how Jesus paid the price for them on the cross. If I come to him with a heart of repentance and a desire to know God by inviting Jesus into my life, God's word says that I have been forgiven, that the price for those sins has been paid in full.

If God remembers my sins no more, then I also have a responsibility to accept that forgiveness and even to forgive myself. Of course, some of the things I've done are harder to forgive than others, and I'll never forget them.

It does help to have a heart full of gratitude to God for his forgiveness of me. It also helps to recognize that everyone—every human being who has ever lived, no matter how good we might perceive a person to be—is in the same boat. That's because there's only been one perfect person: Jesus, our Savior.

Oh, Lord, please give me courage, inspiration, and imagination when I need it. Please heal the hurts in my heart. Help me to accept your forgiveness and to forgive myself. Help me to not retaliate against those who have hurt me. Make me read and breathe the right words through my mind. Give me wisdom and insight—not of my own but such that your word touches me and even flows through me. In Jesus' name, amen.

by Debbie

April 11

Last night an angel of the God to whom I belong and whom I serve stood beside me and said, "Do not be afraid, Paul. You must stand trial before Caesar; and God has graciously given you the lives of all who sail with you." So keep up your courage, men, for I have faith in God that it will happen just as he told me. Nevertheless, we must run aground on some island.
Acts 27:23–26

What struck me about this scripture is how Paul's ship was going to experience shipwreck, but the men should still *take heart.* How many times have we had shipwrecks in our lives and felt that surely doom was all around? Yet God says to *take courage.* The ship may wreck, but you won't be harmed.

I thought about that with our weight-loss journey. We all set sail in different ways. We keep on course. Along the way we kept up. Then for some of us, the ship ran aground. For others, the shipwreck will come. We can't keep on the same course. If we do, the ship will founder. But God tells us to take heart. To reposition ourselves. That we'll reach land, and our health will be much better.

What was the key that them from drowning? Paul listened! He heard God tell him what to do, and he told them. Had they chosen their own way, they would have drowned.

Am I listening? If I do, I'll make it. If I don't, then I'm afraid the news won't be so good. So whether it's weight or life issues right now, I need to take heart. The ship may wreck, but God will see me through.

Father, thank you for telling me what I need to know so that I'll have courage, and I'll be able to take heart and trust in you. In Jesus' name, amen.

by Nancy

April 12

I will give you a new heart and put a new spirit in you;
I will remove from you your heart of stone and give you a heart of flesh.
And I will put my Spirit in you and move you to follow
my decrees and be careful to keep my laws.
Ezekiel 36: 26–27

Even to your old age and gray hairs I am he, I am he who
will sustain you. I have made you and I will carry you;
I will sustain you and I will rescue you.
Isaiah 46:4

I am not an accident. God planned everything about me ahead of time. God says he will take care of me throughout my entire life, even into my old age.

Since I'm often filled with fear instead of faith, that's a good reminder. If God cares for me, he also accepts me. One question to consider, then, is what areas about myself am I still struggling to accept?

My tendency toward introversion, which often leads to isolating? My difficulties with overeating and excess body weight? My fear and self-doubt? I'm beginning to address those things—not in my own power, but by asking God to change me, as I have no power to change myself.

Father, please forgive me for letting fear keep me from doing the things you have asked me to do. Please help me as I move forward and as I seek to do your will. Father, let me not give up on the dreams you have put into my heart. Where I am weak, please be strong for me. Where I procrastinate, give me the motivation to move ahead. Let me do your will always. In Jesus' name, amen.

by Debbie

April 13

The Lord is my light and my salvation—whom shall I fear?
The Lord is the stronghold of my life—of whom shall I be afraid?
Psalm 27:1

I sought the Lord, and he answered me; he delivered me
from all my fears. Those who look to him are radiant;
their faces are never covered with shame.
Psalm 34:4–5

The Lord revealed to me some things about fear.

First, it's a powerful motivator. Fear of the unknown is so hard, and it can drive me to do things that I wouldn't normally do. Or it will paralyze me so I don't do what I need to do.

Fear will also tell me that there's no way I'll lose the weight. No way I'll get that job I need. No way I could help someone in need.

Fear is something that can lead to shame. I know I'm supposed to do something, but fear stopped me. Then I feel bad that I didn't do what I was supposed to. It becomes a vicious circle.

Fear has even protected me. Because of some things that happened in the past, I felt that being overweight would prevent them from happening again. But in reality, the fear is hurting me.

God wants to take that from me. He doesn't want me walking around in fear and shame. God would rather I work through the fears.

Father, show me my fears and then show me what they're doing to my life. Help me to give each of my fears to you. God, help me realize that you'll bring me through anything I need to face. Help me to stand strong and keep the faith. Help me to trust you instead of in my fears. In Jesus' name, amen.

by Nancy

April 14

Now, Lord, consider their threats and enable your servants to speak your word with great boldness.
Acts 4:29

I eagerly expect and hope that I will in no way be ashamed, but will have sufficient courage so that now as always Christ will be exalted in my body, whether by life or by death.
Philippians 1:20

I'm just beginning to learn what it means to live without fear. I'm only partway along that journey, but God is teaching me about boldness. About being willing to proclaim the truth of who he is. About speaking the truth. About standing up for what's right without fear. There is often a price to pay for doing that, and someday I may have to pay it. It may cost me dearly. I may suffer because of it. Am I willing to do that? I'm not sure yet. I hope I could be strong enough, but I won't know until I face it.

In the meantime, I need to have another kind of courage. The courage to say no to myself when it feels like every cell in my body wants to say yes. The courage to turn to God instead of to food. The courage to turn my entire will, my entire life over to God, including the urge to overeat, my favorite foods, and my stubbornness about not wanting to change the way I eat.

If countless believers could face martyrdom for living out their faith, I should be able to do a little thing like giving up sugar, obeying God when he wants me to eat oatmeal for breakfast, or being willing to give up a food I've been holding onto.

Father, give me boldness. Give me courage. Help me to live for you. In Jesus' name, amen.

by Debbie

April 15

And the God of all grace, who called you to his eternal glory in Christ, after you have suffered a little while, will himself restore you and make you strong, firm, and steadfast.
1 Peter 5:10

There are a number of areas in which I excel; keeping track of my things isn't one of them. It's comical really. I receive gifts from my family to help me keep track of things that are easily lost. Alas, lost things are most always found (usually by my wife). As she reunites me with my possessions, I always ask her the same question, "Where was it?"

"Where was it?" This is the most common question we ask when lost things are recovered. We ask because we care. We ask because "loss" is the most painful and familiar consequence of sin. Our sin results in the loss of everything that matters the most to us. Sin robs us of our resources, our relationships, our joy, and our peace. The internal satisfaction associated with FOUNDness is nearly indescribable.

Good Friday is our day to reflect upon what sin has taken from us, and where sin has taken us from. Good Friday is SO GOOD, because on that day, God himself, in the person of Jesus, came all the way into the depths of our sin. He FOUND us. He opened the pathway for us to be restored to our rightful place and personhood. Let's take the time to reflect today. Where did he find you? What has he restored?

Father, every day we need you to recover what we've lost. We need to be found. Encouraged. Renewed. We need YOU. Thank you for what you did for us on the cross so that you could restore your lost ones. Us. In Jesus' name, amen.

by Pastor Chris

April 16

"And why do you worry about clothes? See how the flowers of the field grow. They do not labor or spin. Yet I tell you that not even Solomon in all his splendor was dressed like one of these. If that is how God clothes the grass of the field, which is here today and tomorrow is thrown into the fire, will he not much more clothe you—you of little faith? So do not worry, saying, 'What shall we eat?' or 'What shall we drink?' or 'What shall we wear?' For the pagans run after all these things, and your heavenly Father knows that you need them. But seek first his kingdom and his righteousness, and all these things will be given to you as well. Therefore do not worry about tomorrow, for tomorrow will worry about itself. Each day has enough trouble of its own."
Matthew 6:28–34

My emotions can get the best of me. It can take the smallest thing, and I'm off in a rage or in tears. I can watch a TV competition show and cry. I'll cry if the competitor wins. I'll also cry if they don't do well. On other days I just go with the flow without much bothering me. I wonder why our emotions can be so fickle. Is it body chemistry or circumstances?

My emotions can also determine how well I'll do with my eating or with my level of energy. God really knew what he was talking about when he told us not to worry about tomorrow. I chose this scripture because I need to hear just how much he cares. He'll meet my every need. He'll get me through whatever it is that's going on in my life *right now*. I don't need to worry about it. I don't need to cry. I just need to seek him. Sometimes God doesn't calm the storm. Sometimes he lets the storm rage and calms his child. If I ask him.

Father, to you I give all my emotions and all my tomorrows. In Jesus' name, amen.

by Nancy

April 17

Shallum son of Hallohesh, ruler of a half-district of Jerusalem, repaired the next section with the help of his daughters.
Nehemiah 3:12

The first chapters of Nehemiah are focused on a remnant of Israelites who, having been sent back from exile in the Persian empire, were rebuilding Jerusalem. Studying this passage was part of my effort to read through the entire Bible in a year. In a rote list of which people and families repaired which sections of the city wall, I noticed this small phrase: "with the help of his daughters."

Sometimes when I think of the status of women in Bible times, I forget that God used many women to accomplish his purposes, even in the midst of a highly patriarchal society. Strong women. Women of courage. Women of faith. Women like Sarah, Miriam, Tamar, Rahab, Ruth, Deborah, Abigail, Esther, Mary Magdalene, and Mary the mother of Jesus.

None of these women were perfect, but they did allow God to use them, which makes them my heroes. And here again, in Nehemiah's time, were women who were willing to do what was necessary to do God's will. Reading about them makes me want to be like them. Someday, when we're in God's eternal kingdom together, I would like to meet all those amazing women, including the daughters of Shallum who helped to rebuild a section of the wall of Jerusalem.

Father, thank you for telling the truth about those amazing women, for making them real *so that I know despite my weaknesses that I can strive to be like them. Give me the same kind of faith. The same kind of courage. Help me to be strong like they were. In Jesus' name, amen.*

by Debbie

April 18

But the fruit of the Spirit is love, joy, peace, forbearance,
kindness, goodness, faithfulness, gentleness, and self-control.
Against such things there is no law.
Galatians 5:22–23

I've been thinking a lot about fear. I must admit that I have much fear in my life. For example, I became claustrophobic due to a trauma in my life. And I absolutely hate and fear Asian beetles.

These fears can stem from small things or big things.

Then I have to ask myself, do I fear losing the weight? I think so. Because I was raped when I was younger, in some ways I use the weight as a way to keep men from looking at me. Furthermore, I don't take compliments well. I'm sure that's because I don't want to be noticed. I don't want anyone looking at me. To overcome these fears, I have to focus on what God is saying in the verse above. I can have love, joy, peace, forbearance, kindness, goodness, faithfulness, gentleness, and, yes, even self-control. If I have God's spirit within me, I already have those things.

God doesn't want me to live in a spirit of fear. He wants me to have all those good things, all of the fruit of the spirit. Even if you try to insert the word fear into that verse, it just doesn't fit. It's not at all part of what God wants for me—or for you.

Father, I pray that I can live in the fruit of the spirit that you want to give all of us. Lord, I lay my fear down at your feet. I trust that you will take care of me and that nothing can come against me in this journey of freedom from addiction. Thank you, Father. In Jesus' name, amen.

by Nancy

April 19

"Bring the whole tithe into the storehouse, that there may be food in my house. Test me in this," says the Lord Almighty, "and see if I will not throw open the floodgates of heaven and pour out so much blessing that there will not be room enough to store it."
Malachi 3:10

I pray that out of his glorious riches he may strengthen you with power through his Spirit in your inner being.
Ephesians 3:16

Fear has been one of my prime motivators toward sin. It would not surprise me if that was true for most of us, considering how many times in the Bible, God tells us to "fear not." One of the things I've been afraid of is of not having enough. Enough food. Enough money to live a comfortable life.

With food it wasn't a fear of starving—I've been blessed enough never to have to worry about that. But there was always an urge to eat more than I needed. It seems like nothing ever really filled me up because what I was hungry for wasn't food. The emptyness I felt could only be filled up by Spirit of God.

In this weight-loss journey, I've learned to trust God to meet my material and spiritual needs. I learned to turn to him with my false hunger. In the process I learned that I can't outgive God. If I faithfully give a tithe of my income, he provides everything else. If I turn to him with my compulsion to eat, he answers. He has provided abundantly. And that provision has increased my trust, my faith, and my love for him.

Father, thank you for being there to provide everything I need. Thank you for filling me up when I feel empty. In Jesus' name, amen.

by Debbie

April 20

You must return to the Lord your God with your whole being.
Deuteronomy 30:10 NCV

This verse got my mind whirling. You must RETURN to the Lord your God with your WHOLE BEING! Wow—that means we have left the Lord when we choose to overeat. What a horrible thought. I would never want to leave the Lord.

It goes on to say we must return with our WHOLE BEING! At first that sounded like a lot of work to me! Then I imagined Jesus on the cross. His face was sweating. He just carried that cross, all the while battered and bruised (don't we feel like that sometimes?) and bleeding. He worked hard! He was doing with His WHOLE BEING something for me. He was dying for me! He could have given up and called the angels in. He could have said, "I just can't do this anymore. It is too difficult." But he didn't. He pressed through. He died!

That makes me feel selfish for my little thoughts: *God I'm tired of this. I can't do this anymore.* Those thoughts that are "stinking thinking."

I must remember that HE ROSE! He conquered sin and the grave. Something so awesome it is hard to even put into words came out of that sweat and the work of his WHOLE BEING.

I hate that it will take time for the weight to come off, but I have to keep going. I can't give into the world's mentality of "give it to me now!" I must remember to keep pressing in with my WHOLE BEING! To RETURN to the Lord as of this moment!

Father, give me courage, give me perseverance, help me to press on. In Jesus' name, amen.

by Nancy

April 21

Do not be anxious about anything, but in every situation, by prayer and petition, with thanksgiving, present your requests to God.
Philippians 4:6

For the Spirit God gave us does not make us timid, but gives us power, love, and self-discipline.
2 Timothy 1:7

I was at a meeting once when someone spoke about her "crazy thinking." She shared that she experienced a terrible fear that there would be an earthquake and something would fall down and hit her dog in the head. We were in Southern California, so earthquakes were a "reasonable" fear. Yet expecting it to happen in exactly that way wasn't rational.

I was surprised at how much I related to what she said, because I see myself as a reasonable person. Earlier that day I had experienced a similar fear, out of the blue, about having a horrendous car accident. It probably came on because someone had been following me too closely when I had to stop quickly for a traffic light.

I've never been one to obsess over "what ifs," but it was instructive to hear what she did in response. There's a way to deal with fear without overeating. Food doesn't have to be my go-to when I'm afraid. I can pray, I can write in my journal, I can call someone and ask her to pray with me, and I can share a prayer request among friends on social media or by text. I can do any of those things anytime fear hits me seemingly out of nowhere.

Thank you, God, for always providing a way out of irrational thinking and for reminding me frequently in your word to "fear not." As I learn to trust you more and more, thank you for giving me peace to replace the fear. Amen.

by Debbie

April 22

Finally, be strong in the Lord and in his mighty power. Put on the full armor of God, so that you can take your stand against the devil's schemes.
Ephesians 6:10–11

When I think of a victor, I picture someone with a shield strapped to his arm. A sword in his hand. He's standing over someone—foot firmly planted on his back—shouting victory. The enemy has been defeated. Yet when I think about defeating the evil of obesity, the thought of "going to war" and "fighting" wears me out. I think, *There's no way I can bear the weight of that heavy shield. There's no way I can go out there in my own power and fight.*

Beth Moore, in her *Breaking Free* Bible study, wrote something really thought-provoking: "God wants us to be victors. We don't become victors by conquering the enemy. We become victors through surrender to Christ. We don't become victors by our independence from the enemy. We become victors by our dependence on God. Victorious lives flow from victorious thoughts. Thinking victorious thoughts comes from setting our focus on a victorious God."

I go back to what I've always said: We tend to make things a lot harder than they need to be. We put God in a box. We see him as throwing us out to the wolves as if he were saying, "You're on your own now, go get 'em!" But he never does that. He sticks around and fights our battles for us. Our victory is found *through* him. It's not found in our own hands. He's the only one who can change us. It is in him that we live and breathe.

Jesus, it's by your name that Satan is defeated. Help me remember to speak your name today. Line up my thoughts with yours. Bring me victory in those things I cannot do in my own power. Fight the fight for me. Amen.

by Nancy

April 23

And the word of the Lord came to [Elijah]: "Depart from here and turn eastward and hide yourself by the brook Cherith, which is east of the Jordan. You shall drink from the brook, and I have commanded the ravens to feed you there."
1 Kings 17:2–4 ESV

I participated in a women's Bible study about Elijah by Priscilla Sherer. The first part of the study was on this passage, which shows how—before Elijah had his big Mt. Carmel/bring-down-fire-from-heaven moment—God sent him into the wilderness for an extended time. Not long ago, I experienced this kind of sending away. I left a home and job in Southern California and came to live with my aging mother to help her around the house and with expenses. I arrived without much savings. After six months, I still hadn't found a job. Did I experience fear in the face of that? Yes! Yet God took care of me throughout seven months without a steady income.

I continued to do freelance work and I also received a larger-than-normal tax refund. Somehow, I didn't miss paying any bills, including a substantial car payment. My credit rating stayed the same. And I did something I had never been completely faithful in doing until then: I gave a regular tithe. As I started my weight-loss journey and learned to depend more and more on God, he also taught me to trust him with my finances. I learned to trust that he would meet my needs in all ways—mentally, emotionally, spiritually, and through material provision. I learned that it is God who supplies—just as he did for Elijah so very long ago.

Father, thank you for teaching me that it's you who provides. That I don't need to live in fear of living without. Thank you for your lovingkindness. In Jesus' name, amen.

by Debbie

April 24

If any of you lacks wisdom, you should ask God, who gives generously to all without finding fault, and it will be given to you. But when you ask, you must believe and not doubt, because the one who doubts is like a wave of the sea, blown and tossed by the wind.
James 1:6

I was once watching a reality TV show called *Fat March.* The contestants were interviewed after the show, and one thing that stood out to me was how many of them said how important it was to believe in yourself. How many of us truly believe in ourselves?

They talked about when you doubt that you can do something, believe in yourself and just do it, and you'll find that you'll be able to do that and even more. Many of them had a hard time walking a mile. And by the time the show was over, they had walked more than five hundred.

There is truth in that message. If we lack faith in ourselves, we'll fail. Even God says that doubt is like a crashing wave.

I know I am going to start with some positive self-talk. I'm going to start by believing that I can get those last pounds off. I'm going to believe that I can go all day without a snack. That I can go all day with a set amount of food and no more.

That makes me think of the song by Martina McBride, "Anyway." The lyrics are a good reminder: "Do it anyway." Even when it's tough. In addition to encouraging others, I need to take time each day to encourage myself. To build myself up. To get the negative talk out of my language. To believe in myself!

Father, your word encourages me. In the same way, let me not speak discouragement to myself, but courage instead. In Jesus' name, amen.

by Nancy

April 25

I will praise the Lord, who counsels me; even at night my heart instructs me. I keep my eyes always on the Lord. With him at my right hand, I will not be shaken.
Psalm 16:7–8

I have heard this again and again from other overeaters like me: I have the most trouble with wanting to eat at night. Sometimes it's all evening long. Sometimes it's just late at night. I've heard people talk about waking up in the middle of the night wanting to eat. I have the same problem. There's something about sitting down at night after dinner, relaxing, watching TV, or doing something else as I'm winding down from a day of work (or when I was a young mom, after a day spent caring for my kids) that makes me want to turn to my favorite comfort: food.

I can usually do well most of the day. And then something tends to break down at night. Maybe it's because I've let down my guard. Or the day's problems are wearing on me. Or I'm just plain weary. If I'm in that position, I'm at my most vulnerable to reaching for my go-to comfort, usually something sweet.

That's why I was so happy to see this verse in Psalm 16: "the Lord who counsels me; even *at night* my heart instructs me." That is such a blessing, knowing that God knows my struggles, and he's willing to counsel me about what to do when I'm basically defenseless. If I remember to turn to him and ask (I don't always remember to do that) he'll provide a way out. He'll remind me to drink some water. Call a friend. Read his word. Listen to music. Sing a song. Have courage. I don't have to eat to feel better. It's in turning to him that I can find my victory.

Father, thank you for always being there when I need you. Amen.

by Debbie

April 26

What goes into someone's mouth does not defile them, but what comes out of their mouth, that is what defiles them.
Matthew 15:11

What do we say about ourselves? Are they words that will encourage us, or are they words that will tear us down?

My mouth has so much power. I have the power in my tongue to succeed at whatever I need to in life. If I need to lose weight, are my words lining up with that? Am I reminding myself about who I am in Christ? Or am I beating myself down?

Many times, I have stepped on the scale, and the foulest things have come out of my mouth. I would never ever want to hear anyone being called the things I call myself.

But I wonder . . . if I turned that around and chose words of encouragement, would that help? Would losing weight become a bit easier?

I do know this for sure: When I beat myself down, it doesn't encourage me. In fact, many times I have said to myself, "You'll always be a fat pig." What if instead I said, "God loves me as I am. I know that he wants me healthy. So onward I go."

Which one felt better as you read it?

It's so easy to think negative thoughts. But I can train my brain to come up with healthy, encouraging thoughts instead. And it will be worth it. God says I'm worth it.

Father, part of the word "encourage" is "courage." Give me courage from encouraging words. Help me not to discourage myself with demoralizing thoughts and words. If I forget and tell myself something bad, remind me quickly to take it back. And thank you for the encouraging words I find in scripture. In Jesus' name, amen.

by Nancy

April 27

So will My word be which goes out of My mouth;
It will not return to Me empty, without accomplishing what I desire,
and without succeeding in the purpose for which I sent it.
Isaiah 55:11

How do I know that I can trust God? The first way I know it is to know his word in the Bible. If I look throughout scripture, I see a unity of purpose and a unity of message. I see that over and over again as God kept his promises. I know that I can trust a promise keeper. I know he'll do what he promises me.

Another way is to remember those things he has done in my life. How he first brought me to belief in him. How he has provided for me and met all my needs. How he has given me things above and beyond what I've been able even to imagine.

A third way is to listen to the testimony of others for whom God has done great things. I think of so many Old Testament heroes. My favorites are Joseph, an intelligent man who wholeheartedly trusted God; David, a man after God's own heart; Elijah, who was obedient and bold; and Esther, who overcame her fears.

It's important to trust that God will do for me what I cannot do for myself. When I have trust in God, then I can be bold, even when I'm afraid. I can step forward in faith. I can obey even when it's difficult, because I know that God will bring me through whatever circumstance he has put me in. Even the hard ones. The ones that aren't so fun. The ones that test my patience. The ones that I'm afraid of. The ones that hurt.

I can do all things through Christ, who strengthens me.

Father, you know that I'm naturally weak and timid. It is only through you that I can be bold. Give me courage. Help me to be bold in you. Amen.

by Debbie

April 28

"Not by might nor by power, but by my Spirit," says the Lord Almighty.
Zechariah 4:6

How many times, especially as I have read stories from the Old Testament, have I seen God take weak people and use them to demonstrate his power? So many that I'm sure I can't name them all. Moses, David, Gideon, Elijah, Esther. So many more. Moses had a speech impediment when God asked him to free the Israelites, David was just a boy when he faced Goliath, God asked Gideon to stand down most of his army and go out to battle with just three hundred men, Elijah was afraid of Jezebel's threats, despite just having called down fire from heaven, and Esther was afraid of being executed should her husband, the king, find out she was Jewish. God used them all to accomplish great—and often impossible—things, according to his purposes.

If God can work through those weak people, he can work in and through this weak vessel too. So—how can God help me to overcome my addictive behavior around food? "Not by might nor by power, but by my Spirit," says the Lord Almighty.

The same power is available to me every day as I face my own giants and impossible situations. The same power that parted the Red Sea. The same power that won the battle for Gideon's men. The same power that raised Jesus from the dead. One of those impossible situations, of course, is my struggle with overeating. Yet if I choose to lean on God's power and strength rather than trying to do it on my own, I have the whole of heaven's power behind me. I just have to want to and . . . ask.

Father, give me your power in the midst of my great weakness. In Jesus' name, amen.

by Debbie

April 29

Therefore, if anyone is in Christ, he is a new creation.
The old has passed away; behold, the new has come.
2 Corinthians 5:17

I did some planting for my mom and mother-in-law. I was thinking that some of the plants looked pretty pathetic. Not the prettiest. Like they were barely hanging on. But I knew within a few weeks they were going to grow to be beautiful, and some would produce some really good food.

Sometimes plants like those have to weather the storms. The wind and rain. Yet they come out beautifully. They may wither for a day or two with the heat, but they come back with just a little bit of water. With just a little encouragement, they bounce right back. Sometimes it's the same way with us. The storms come and we slip a bit, but with just a little encouragement we can make it through as we wait for sunnier days.

It's the same with butterflies. They're not so cute in the beginning, but look how they turn out. They really are beautiful. Their colors are gorgeous. They go through quite a bit to get to that point, but the end result is spectacular.

So here is your encouragement: You can do this. You can make it through this journey. You can live your life to the fullest. You've got this! You are *awesome*, and you are *beautiful.*

Father, thank you so much for your promises. Thank you that I know that I can do this when you throw your strength behind me, when you fight for me. You are my encourager and my strength. I hold on tight to you as I look forward to better days ahead. In Jesus' name, amen.

by Nancy

April 30

And my God will meet all your needs
according to the riches of his glory in Christ Jesus.
Philippians 4:19

One of the things I've realized over time is that part of the reason I overeat is a fear of not getting enough. I'm not even sure why I feel that way. It isn't because I've ever truly gone hungry, but for some reason the fear is there just the same.

This is especially true at night. I allow myself a small snack in the evening as long as I haven't yet reached my calorie limit for the day. If I have, though, I shouldn't need a snack. And yet I have often felt fear—what if I get hungry again before bedtime? What if I can't make it through the rest of the evening without a snack (even though I shouldn't physically need one)?

Part of what I have had to do is to pray about it. Many of my prayers go like this: "Jesus, please make what I've already eaten today be enough." Or "Jesus, let me make it through till morning without needing to eat anything else."

The truth I've had to face in all this is that my body needs far less food than I sometimes think it needs. My body only needs an amount of food that will maintain my health and a healthy body weight. Anything more is overeating.

That means that if my mind and emotions tell me that I need more, then somehow my brain and my feelings are lying to me. There is a remedy to that, though: trust in God. And trusting in God means surrendering my food to him, no matter what.

Father, you know what my body needs. Give me the courage to recognize that truth as well. Build my trust in you so that I listen to you rather than to my own imperfect feelings. In Jesus' name, Amen.

by Debbie

Cry of Our Hearts

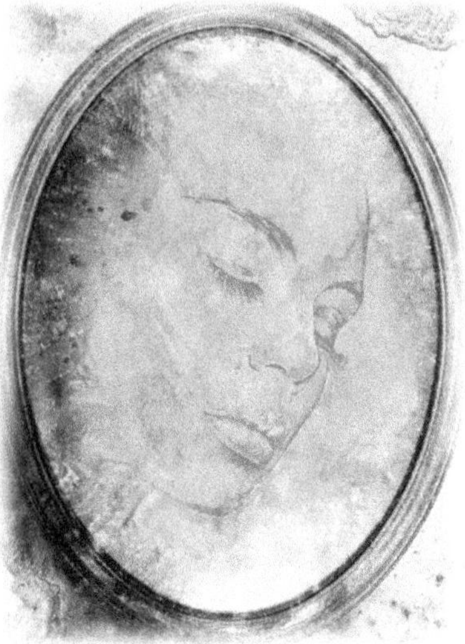

INTEGRITY

We recognize the power of confessing the truth.

CRY OF OUR HEARTS

May 1

But your iniquities have separated you from your God;
your sins have hidden his face from you, so that he will not hear.
Isaiah 59:2

Whoever conceals his transgressions will not prosper,
but he who confesses and forsakes them will obtain mercy.
Proverbs 28:13 ESV

One of the ways I can walk in integrity in my life is by confessing my sins. To God. And to another human being. There's a saying you'll hear in twelve-step programs: "You're only as sick as your secrets." There's something to be said about being honest about our failings (in the appropriate context, of course).

Being open about what's wrong in my life makes me real. It takes away the false ideal of perfectionism. It shows that it's God who makes the way out of my weakness, that I can't do it on my own strength. It means I don't blame other people for my own failings. All of those things keep me humble.

It means I should boast about what God has done for me rather than what I've done for myself. That doesn't mean I can't be proud of my accomplishments; I can. There are many things I've worked hard for. But it also helps me recognize that I can't truly accomplish anything alone. I need God's help, and most of the time I need the help of other people as well.

Confessing my sins also makes me more grateful. And it ensures that God will cleanse me "from all unrighteousness."

Father, thank you for showing me how important it is to confess my sins. When I've done something wrong, please remind me to get it off my chest quickly, so I can ask for (and receive) your forgiveness. In Jesus name, amen.

by Debbie

May 2

If we confess our sins, he is faithful and just and will forgive us our sins and purify us from all unrighteousness.
1 John 1:9

One thing that unconfessed sin does is that it isolates me. Think of what happened in the Garden of Eden at the fall of man; once Adam and Eve had sinned by eating the forbidden fruit, they hid from God. But they also covered themselves with fig leaves because they were ashamed, and that was a way of hiding from each other.

We were not meant to live in isolation. God made us social beings. We need each other. This is especially true for people who are trying to overcome an addiction, such as compulsive overeating. It helps immensely knowing that there's someone out there who understands my struggle. Someone who knows what I mean when I talk about wrestling with nighttime eating or scarfing down six donuts at one sitting because I couldn't stop or hiding sweets around the house that I then ate in secret.

But once I confess my sins, I no longer have anything to hide. And when I don't have anything to hide, I no longer need to hide from people. In that way, I can walk through life with integrity. That's freedom! It's secrecy that kept me in bondage to my sin. But when I confessed it, the shackles were broken. It no longer has the power to hold me, bring me down, and keep me addicted, a slave to whatever it was that I was chained to every day of my life. For me that was the compulsion to overeat.

Father, never let me forget that I'm only as sick as my secrets. Show me the importance of confessing my sins—not just to you, but to friends who can hold me accountable. Thank you for your mercy and forgiveness. In Jesus' name, amen.

by Debbie

May 3

Do not lie to each other, since you have taken off your old self with its practices, and have put on the new self, which is being renewed in knowledge in the image of its Creator.
Colossians 3:9–10

In one sermon our pastor talked about lying and having integrity. He also talked about wearing masks. That made me think. How honest am I with myself about my eating? My habits?

When I count calories, that opens my eyes to just how much I eat and how I'm eating so many wrong things. My biggest problem is not so much the volume as the stuff I eat. And the snacks. I often eat out of boredom. I've also always thought that I don't want to hide my eating from anyone, and if I got to that point, then I'd know I had crossed a line. So I've been forthcoming about my eating. Until recently. I found myself doing the dishes after my nighttime snack and making sure they were put away before my husband could see the dishes in the morning. That opened my eyes to ask myself, *how honest am I?* The only person I'm hurting by my dishonesty is me.

God's word tells us that we've taken off the old and put on the new. When I pray and ask God to take this from me, I'm putting on the new. Now it's up to me if I'm going to stain my new self. He'll keep renewing me, but I have to be willing to let him. I have to put off the dishonesty. The pride. And humble myself before the Lord. Let him create something new and awesome in me.

Father, I ask that you would renew my spirit. Renew my mind. Help me overcome this addiction, these destructive habits. Create a new, healthier version of me. Help me become more and more like you. Thank you, Lord. In Jesus' name, amen.

by Nancy

May 4

The one who is faithful in a very little thing is also faithful in much; and the one who is unrighteous in a very little thing is also unrighteous in much.
Luke 16:10

Merriam-Webster defines the word "integrity" as follows: 1: a firm adherence to a code of especially moral or artistic values: incorruptibility. 2: an unimpaired condition: soundness. 3: the quality or state of being complete or undivided: completeness. It's clear that integrity is much more than just being honest with myself. It implies authenticity, purity, and wholeness. In biblical terms, you might think of the word "righteousness."

It's also clear that I can't have integrity based on my own power. Why? Because only God is good. God has chosen to construct the universe so that I have no choice but to depend on him in order to be able to meet his standard, which is perfection. I know I can't be perfect, so what, then, am I supposed to do? I have to turn to the One who is perfect and ask him to give me his righteousness, his integrity, and his ability to overcome my weaknesses (which the Bible calls "the flesh" and "sin").

God made a way. He sent his Son, Jesus, to pay the price for my weakness and sin. To make a way so that I can have victory over them. Of course, I won't be perfect as long as I'm in this weak vessel of a body—that will come later (God has promised). But I can overcome my compulsive overeating. If I'm willing. If I hand my will over to him. If I surrender.

Then I might, through God's grace and mercy, have the power to walk in integrity.

Father, thank you for what you did by sending your Son to save us. Help me now as I seek to walk in integrity rather than in weakness. Amen.

by Debbie

May 5

This is what the Lord says:
"When people fall down, do they not get up?
When someone turns away, do they not return?"
Jeremiah 8:4

In this scripture, the Lord is remonstrating with his people for not turning away from their wicked ways. He's saying: "Isn't it obvious that when someone falls down that they automatically get up again?" But it wasn't obvious to the Israelites. They continued in their idolatry, and the Lord eventually punished them.

In this weight-loss journey, in my recovery from addiction, I haven't perfectly adhered to any principle or plan. I've been a weak human being. I've given in to cravings, and I have overeaten at times. I have gone back to eating foods that I already know are troublesome (i.e., addictive) for me.

In the past, when I failed, I often used it as an excuse to give up entirely. But this journey has been different. Each time I have failed, I've seen it as *information.* I examine what happened and ask myself: "What can I learn from this?" If I truly understand and learn from my mistake, I can ask the Lord to help me not to do it again. I need to ALWAYS remember that failure is not the opposite of success; it's part of success. Failure is not a loss, but a gain that allows me to learn, change, and grow. If I recognize that truth instead of using my failure as an excuse to rebel, then when I fall, I can get right back up and try again tomorrow.

Father, thank you for helping me back up again when I fall. When I fail, help me remember that you are merciful and gracious, always willing to forgive and even forget. Help me to walk in integrity, always keeping my eyes on the prize ahead. In Jesus' name, amen.

by Debbie

May 6

The one who is faithful in a very little thing is also faithful in much; and the one who is unrighteous in a very little thing is also unrighteous in much.
Luke 16:10

When I quit smoking, one of the steps that God had to take me through was to find all the scriptures showing how much of a sin that was in my life. It was painful to realize how sinful I was being, but that knowledge brought freedom.

The Lord has been talking to me to do the same thing with my eating. He let me see how easy it is to say "Lord, forgive me" and not really mean it. To not really realize how big of a sin it is! I need to see that, because I'm really not one who likes to make the Lord weep. But I believe he does. I know he does.

I had been taught that the Lord doesn't have emotions, so I never pictured the Lord weeping until one Sunday during worship our pastor's wife asked me to come forward because the Lord had something to say to me. The word from the Lord was that he had cried each time I had a child die. He wept each time I was hurting from the death of a child. There was not a dry eye in the place. And I got to see God's heart that day.

Now I realize that God also weeps over my disobedience. No, he's not angry with me, but I believe it hurts him to watch it. We cry when our kids do hurtful things, and God's love is so much greater than ours. Why would I think he wouldn't be hurt? Yet I don't ever want to be the reason for him to cry.

Father, give me the integrity to not be two-faced with my sin. Help me to always remember that you weep over it—not because it hurts you, but because you love me and you know it hurts me. In Jesus' name, amen.

by Nancy

May 7

I will be careful to lead a blameless life—when will you come to me?
I will conduct the affairs of my house with a blameless heart.
Psalm 101:2

If I look through the scriptures, I find that there were a few people who really did live blameless lives. They had integrity. They were the same in private as they were in public. They chose to do what was right even when no one was looking. Mary, the mother of Jesus, was one. Job was another. Were they perfect? Of course not—there was only one perfectly sinless person who walked the earth, and he became the Savior of the world.

But with God's help, I can live and walk in integrity. And if I haven't done so in the past, I can start now. I can start with a self-examination, asking God to show me what I've done wrong and who I've wronged. I can make restitution or make amends whenever and wherever I can. I can stop doing those things that are contrary to God's word and his will for my life.

One way I can live in integrity is to stop living a double life with my food. I can stop keeping a special stash of food, and I can stop eating in secret. I can choose a specific amount of food to eat each day and certain foods that I agree to abstain from. I can stick to that plan to the best of my ability. I can weigh and measure my food, which keeps me honest. I can log my food into a food diary (I use a phone app) to keep myself on the straight and narrow. I can promise myself and God that I won't fudge on amounts. I can choose to live with integrity with my food. And I can ask God to help me do it.

Father, give me a heart that longs to walk in integrity, that desires true honesty, that longs to do what is right in your eyes. In Jesus name, amen.

by Debbie

May 8

In the beginning was the Word, and the Word was with God, and the Word was God.
John 1:1

I'm always amazed at the power of words. I'm thankful for them, as I've been an avid reader most of my life. I recently was rereading a Christian fiction series and found myself tearing up at the description of the death of one of the main characters—a martyr's death. I wept, even knowing that this person wasn't real, she was entirely a construct of the author's imagination. And yet what the character "experienced" was real. There have been countless martyrs for the faith who have actually suffered what the author described.

The benefit of reading that bit of fiction was that it reminded me of the importance of keeping an eternal perspective. How often the trivialities of daily life consume my attention! I need to take care of business, but not at the expense of keeping the right perspective about life. Charles E. Hummel, one of the heads of Intervarsity Christian Fellowship, once wrote: "Your greatest danger is letting the urgent things crowd out the important."

This is true even with my weight-loss journey. It helps to remember that my focus should be on what is important, what lasts, and what is eternal. Though I need to face each day as it comes, I also need to remember that my daily choices have eternal consequences. My thoughts, my choices, and my words—whether they're careless or careful—they all matter.

Father, let the words of my mouth and the meditations of my heart be acceptable in your sight. Help me maintain a balance between doing what I need to do today and keeping an eternal perspective. In Jesus' name, amen.

by Debbie

May 9

One who conceals his wrongdoings will not prosper,
but one who confesses and abandons them will find compassion.
Proverbs 28:13 NASB

Owning my mistakes. That's a tough one. If I have to own my mistakes, then I have to admit to having a problem. It means I have to admit that somewhere along the line I made bad choices. I have to admit that I screwed up.

But the good news is that once I own my mistakes, I can ask God to change me. I can take the next step to complete recovery. And I can finally, once and for all, forgive myself.

Do I need to come to the realization that I didn't need that extra bite yesterday? Maybe that candy bar was not such a great idea? And that soda pop—could I have survived the day without it?

I've also been thinking about quantities. That reminded me of the Israelites who wandered in the desert for forty years. When they needed food, God sent them just what they needed. No more. No less. They were to scoop up only the amount they would need for one day. If they took more, it was spoiled by morning.

How has all that overeating spoiled my life? With bad health. In relationships. I think of the lost time with my kids because I didn't have the energy to do things with them. Not being able to do more with my husband. The extra weight affects all parts of our lives, including the spiritual.

Lord, to make things right with you, I confess my sins. Cleanse me from all unrighteousness. Give me a fresh start. Then, help me to take only what I need right now. No more. No less. Help what I eat to be enough, so that I don't need to go back for more. So that I don't want to. In Jesus' name, amen.

by Nancy

May 10

Let your eyes look straight ahead; fix your gaze directly before you. Give careful thought to the paths for your feet and be steadfast in all your ways. Do not turn to the right or the left; keep your foot from evil.
Proverbs 4:25–27

Do I recognize that overeating is a sin? If I think of it in terms of hurting others, hurting me, and that overeating and an obsession with food are idols that block my relationship with God, then I have to say yes, it is a sin. How, then, do I "keep my foot from evil," keep myself from overeating?

One obstacle to achieving this is that even though our culture looks down on fat people, it not only tolerates overeating—it *encourages* it. This is especially true in the church. Food is also integral to cultural celebrations. I mean, how can you celebrate a birthday without cake? Christmas without cookies? Easter without chocolate? The truth is—I can and I do. So can anyone.

When it comes to what I choose to put in my mouth, I have no excuse. I think of vegetarians who choose to not eat meat. I think of Jews who choose to eat kosher. I think of the prophet Daniel, who chose not to eat from the king's table, because it violated the dietary laws he wanted to honor. He chose to oppose the values of the surrounding culture. Why can't I? The truth is—I can if I want to do what is right before God.

When someone offers me something with sugar in it, I refuse. Sometimes people will press because they don't understand. My response? "I can't; I'm allergic," which I believe is true. I make those choices not only because they're the best thing for me, but also because they honor God. And I ask God to give me the strength.

Father, help me to continue to walk in integrity with my food. Amen.

by Debbie

May 11

And we all, who with unveiled faces contemplate the Lord's glory, are being transformed into his image with ever-increasing glory, which comes from the Lord, who is the Spirit.
2 Corinthians 3:18

Before I could change, I had to face the truth about myself. I had to accept it. I had to look at myself as I truly am. I had to recognize that I am someone who is rebellious and full of self-will, especially when it comes to food. I'm someone who, even in my Christian walk, had sins that I had never faced or asked the Lord to remove.

I had to accept that I was a weak human being. That I was full of fear. That I wanted what I wanted when I wanted it and that I didn't care that God wanted something better for me.

When I get stuck in my weight-loss journey, if the scale doesn't move or if I'm going in the wrong direction—if my food is out of control or if my clothes are suddenly getting tighter—it's almost always because there's some hidden sin in me that I haven't faced and that I haven't allowed God to deal with.

In this weight-loss journey, my frequent prayer has to be the same as King David's when he had sinned: "Search me, God, and know my heart; test me and know my anxious thoughts. See if there is any offensive way in me and lead me in the way everlasting" (Psalm 139:23–24).

There are several keys to overcoming compulsive eating, and two of them are acknowledgment and acceptance.

Father, tell me when I've gone down the wrong path, when I've sinned against you, others, or even myself. Then remind me that I need to repent and help me turn around and go the other direction. In Jesus' name, amen.

by Debbie

May 12

Lord, who may dwell in your sacred tent? Who may live on your holy mountain? The one whose walk is blameless, who does what is righteous, who speaks the truth from their heart.
Psalm 15:2

Talk talk talk! That seems to be all I've done over the last fifteen years of my life. I've talked about what I'm going to do to get the weight off. I've talked about what my goal weight should be. I've talked about what I'll give up. I've talked about what I'll eat. I've talked about how much I'm going to exercise. I've talked, talked, talked. And where has all that talk got me? Tired. Emotionally tired. So tired I don't want to talk about it anymore. I want to bury it. I want to be done with it.

So maybe the way to be done with it is to quit talking. Maybe it's time to actually do! It's time to quit the complaining about how hard it is. It's time to quit the excuse: "But God hasn't shown me how to do it yet." It's time to stop lying to myself. It's time to get tough with myself. It's time to wake up. It's time to put actions to the words that have worn me out.

There have been others who have gone before me and lost tons of weight. It's not a new concept. This is real life. This has got to happen for my own health—spiritual and physical.

I mean how true am I being to God and to myself when all I do is talk and not follow through?

So it's time to quit talking. Time to quit hiding behind the fat and move!

Father, help me to stop promising myself with empty words and instead to have the integrity to take that first step out in faith to do what you want me to do. To eat the way you want me to eat. In Jesus' name, amen.

by Nancy

May 13

I will not violate my covenant or alter what my lips have uttered.
Psalm 89:34

There's an old saying that we should bring back into popularity in our culture: "My word is my bond." I practice that kind of integrity in many areas: with my family and in my work. With my friends and with fellow believers. I keep my word as much as possible so that the people in my life know they can trust me.

Where I have fallen down is with food. How many times have I broken a promise to myself about eating? Why do I do that? Why do I allow that kind of self-indulgence to outweigh (no pun intended) my integrity with myself? Or with God?

Is there something different about food? There has to be, because for overeaters like me, it's hard to even imagine that there are people who practice discipline in their food choices and amounts. Yes, amazingly enough, there are actually people out there who do that! If they can, why can't I? Or maybe there's something different about *me.*

One thing I do know from years of reading scripture is that God has set a perfect example in this area. God has integrity. His word is his bond. If he makes a promise, he keeps it. He has made many promises and has already kept many of them. Those that he hasn't yet kept he will keep in the future. What does that mean for me? That I can trust God and that his word is true. I want to be like *him.* I can ask God, who embodies the word "integrity," to help me also act with integrity around food, even when I can't do so alone.

Father, help me to keep my word about my food—to you and to myself. In Jesus' name, amen.

by Debbie

May 14

For by one sacrifice he has made perfect forever
those who are being made holy.
Hebrews 10:14

"Come to me, all you who are weary and burdened, and I will give you rest. Take my yoke upon you and learn from me, for I am gentle and humble in heart, and you will find rest for your souls. For my yoke is easy and my burden is light."
Matthew 11:28-30

At first glance these two scriptures seem not to relate to one another. After all, what does holiness (perfection) have to do with gentleness and a light burden? Aren't those ideas contradictory? No. In Hebrews, it is God who has made us perfect in *position* with him—not that we actually are perfect yet. Notice how the next part of the sentence says that he is *making* us holy, not that we *are* holy.

So how can we be perfect and still not be completely holy? The perfection is in how God sees us based on the sacrifice of Jesus on the cross. Because of Jesus we are perfect, not because of who we are or what we're doing, but because of what Jesus *has done.* That's a great relief. It shows me God's mercy and his unmerited favor toward me.

It's even more of a relief as I think about the topic of integrity—which is the most difficult of all the subjects in this book to write about. Integrity speaks of holiness, of perfection, and I am neither of those things. I still don't eat perfectly. I still sometimes over-indulge. I sometimes get stuck in a holding pattern in my weight loss. There's a phrase for that: "Progress, not perfection."

Father, thank you that you don't expect me to be perfect. Amen.

by Debbie

May 15

You will again have compassion on us; you will tread our sins underfoot and hurl all our iniquities into the depths of the sea.
Micah 7:19

"My bad!" Have you ever heard that saying? I have realized just how much I hate that expression. My kids used to say it a lot, and it just grated on me to no end.

See, I think it sounds a lot like "I'm bad." And I don't think that's really what you mean to say. It's like you're telling people you're bad. So what if people start confessing that yes, you're bad? Is that how you want to go through life?

There is power in the tongue. I know some people argue, "Oh, don't be so literal, it's just a saying." Yet God tells us there is the power of life and death in what we say. If we say "my bad," is that speaking life or death?

Sometimes that thought, "my bad," can come from hearing it as a child. Or even hearing it as an adult. Another saying that's hard for me to hear is "Shame on you." Okay, are we being literal again? Or is there power in the tongue? What are we putting on people and ourselves when we talk like that?

We are *not* bad. Though we *are* sinners, we're also redeemable. We're worth saving. We're children of the King. We don't need to walk around in shame. We're blood-bought children of the Father. We have been redeemed. If we know Jesus, we have been set free from shame and from the sins of the past. And our words about ourselves and about others should reflect that.

Lord God, King of the Universe, remind me that my words are important. Help me to confess what's true and avoid saying things that are not true. In Jesus' name, amen.

by Nancy

May 16

As iron sharpens iron, so one person sharpens another.
Proverbs 27:17

Therefore each of you must put off falsehood and speak truthfully to your neighbor, for we are all members of one body.
Ephesians 4:25

One of the ways I walk in integrity with my weight-loss journey is through accountability. I need to be accountable to God, to others, and to myself.

I'm always accountable to God. Sometimes I try to pretend that he doesn't see, but that's a ridiculous thought, isn't it? It's part of the fall of mankind in Eden—we still try to hide. I can make myself more aware of my accountability to him through daily prayer and Bible study.

I can also make myself accountable to others. There are many ways I could accomplish that, but I choose to do it by attending twelve-step meetings and by making myself accountable to others who also attend those meetings.

One way I'm accountable to myself is by logging all my food into a phone app. Another is to weigh and measure my food (except veggies, which no one has ever accused me of overeating). I also weigh myself, but only once a month so that I won't become obsessed with the numbers on a scale.

Being accountable helps me keep my integrity around my food.

Father, don't let me ever forget how important it is to be accountable to you, to others, and to myself. In Jesus' name, amen.

by Debbie

May 17

Repent, then, and turn to God, so that your sins may be wiped out, that times of refreshing may come from the Lord.
Acts 3:19

One of the profound truths I've learned on this weight-loss journey is that it's not really about the weight. It's about what's going on in my life that's making me eat too much. It's often about the defects in my character that I'm actively ignoring. I've heard it put this way: It's not what you're eating, it's what's eating you. And what's eating me could be any of a multitude of things. Childhood hurts. The inability to forgive someone. Anger. Resentment. Frustration. And a really big one: unconfessed sin.

Before I can confess my sin, though, I have to recognize it. I have no choice but to admit it to myself. I have to stop excusing it. I need to see how serious it is.

One of the ways I can see the gravity of my own sin is to recognize what it does: It blocks my relationship with God and often blocks my relationships with other people. It can keep me from hearing from God. It may keep me from receiving his blessing. And it can certainly throw a monkey wrench into the workings of my personal relationships.

Am I blocking those "times of refreshing from the Lord" by not confessing something that God sees as sin? And I really want that refreshing. So I'd better do something about it. I'd better ask God to show me my sin, I need to confess it, and I need to repent.

Father, open my eyes to the truth. Make me aware of my sin. Help me see how serious it is. I repent of it now. I ask that your mercy and grace would cover it. Then, I pray, refresh my spirit and walk with me again. In Jesus' name, amen.

by Debbie

May 18

How can you say to your brother, "Let me take the speck out of your eye," when all the time there is a plank in your own eye? You hypocrite, first take the plank out of your own eye.
Matthew 7:4–5

I've been thinking about how quick I am to see what everyone else is doing wrong. When it comes to my kids or my husband, I get after them for each little thing. It doesn't matter that it's something small—I just want to keep them "holy."

Isn't it funny how I understand that the Bible says we're not to judge, but then I mentally add "outside my home." Why do I feel I can put legalistic restrictions on my family? I can point out each wrong to them. But I don't think that's how God sees it.

Now I'm not saying we're not to direct and discipline our children. We should. But I also have a tendency to go overboard at times. I have even caught myself thinking, "If they keep that up, they won't see heaven." What a sad attitude for me to have.

One day the Lord showed me that I'd better take my eyes off the speck in my family's eyes and put my attention on the plank in my own. Yes, you guessed it, on the disobedience with my diet.

I cannot in good conscious judge what others do when I can't even tame what I'm doing in my own life. God says that no sin is worse than the other. How many times have I said, "I just don't have time for liars"? Yet I have time for my gluttony? I have time for my selfishness?

Judge not lest you be not judged. Whew! Guess I better watch it!

Father, give me the integrity not to be a hypocrite, to let you deal with my sin first. In Jesus' name, amen.

by Nancy

May 19

And when you stand praying, if you hold anything against anyone, forgive them, so that your Father in heaven may forgive you your sins.
Mark 11:25

I generally don't think of myself as an unforgiving person. I believe that's true. But I'm also someone who used food to suppress my feelings for so many years that I also know that sometimes there are things I hold onto that I'm completely unaware of. And God has had to reveal them to me.

I had a good childhood, but even then I had to forgive my parents for not being perfect (just as my kids have had to do the same for me). I've had to forgive long-ago romantic partners for hurting and even betraying me. I've had to forgive a whole family who introduced two of my kids to drugs, among other things, when they were teens (that's been the most difficult so far, because the consequences have been so great).

If you're married, your marriage is unlikely to last a lifetime unless you can learn to forgive your spouse (frequently). And if you want to successfully stop overeating compulsively, you'll need to put aside your resentments and unforgiveness. You'll have to let go of your anger. Even if you're righteous in your anger, you still need to release it. If you don't, you'll end up turning back to food for comfort again and again.

So I made a list of people who had harmed me, and I spoke their names, and I forgave them. I let my anger go. I let them go. The burden I was carrying was lifted, and I was suddenly free.

Father, if I'm unaware, bring to mind those I need to forgive. If I know who they are but it's hard for me to do it because I'm still hurt and angry, give me the willingness to forgive. In Jesus' name, amen.

by Debbie

May 20

Examine yourselves, to see whether you are in the faith. Test yourselves. Or do you not realize this about yourselves, that Jesus Christ is in you? —unless indeed you fail to meet the test!
2 Corinthians 13:5

One of the things I've been learning about God's true character is his holiness. His perfection. His justice. When faced with perfection, in looking at myself in comparison, I realize how much I fall short. But we wouldn't want him to be any other way. If he wasn't perfect, if he wasn't completely just, if his standard wasn't perfection, then we would be able to complain about him. As it is now, we have nothing to complain about. Not if we believe that he is working everything out for the ultimate good, and I believe that he is. It's what scripture teaches.

The other part of God's character, the one most of us are more familiar with, is his love. And it's through his perfect love that he has made a way for us to also stand before his holy perfection and justice without incurring his fearsome, righteous anger about our sin. That Way is the person of his Son, Jesus.

One thing I've learned in this weight-loss journey is self-examination. And God teaches me more about my imperfect character the more I look at myself. That forces me to acknowledge my weakness and look to God for strength. It forces me to acknowledge my willfulness and repent of it, asking only for knowledge of God's will and the power to carry it out. I'm sure there are people who have been able to overcome addiction in other ways, but I'm not one of them. My addiction to compulsive eating requires me to walk in integrity, with and for God.

Father, help me to understand your holiness; make me holy too. Amen.

by Debbie

May 21

But mark this: There will be terrible times in the last days. People will be lovers of themselves, lovers of money, boastful, proud, abusive, disobedient to their parents, ungrateful, unholy, without love, unforgiving, slanderous, without self-control, brutal, not lovers of the good, treacherous, rash, conceited, lovers of pleasure rather than lovers of God—having a form of godliness but denying its power. Have nothing to do with such people.
2 Timothy 3:1–5

I need to be real with the Lord. Words are words. But words from the heart are what matters. This is not the time to mess around. This is also not the time to judge. People are hurting. People want the authentic. They don't only need the "Thus says the Lord," they also need understanding: "I'm so sorry you're hurting. I have no words for you, but I can pray." We never know what other people have experienced or what they're going through at that moment.

I heard a pastor once say that he was upset by a speeding car. He was judgmental. He discovered later that the driver was going to the hospital to say goodbye to his mother before she passed. Perhaps like him, my first instinct would have been to wish that a cop would come along and pull over that car. But God listens to the heart. He doesn't just listen to my words.

Where is your heart right now? Is it cold? Bitter? Hurting? There's Someone who wants to help. He wants his children to climb in the river and lay bare their souls. Lay out their hurts and struggles. Be authentic with God. Live with integrity! He loves us and wants to be there for us. He wants to build us up and make us stronger.

Father, help me to walk in authenticity and integrity with you. In Jesus' name, amen.

by Nancy

May 22

Who may ascend the mountain of the Lord?
Who may stand in his holy place?
The one who has clean hands and a pure heart,
who does not trust in an idol or swear by a false god.
Psalm 24:3–4

I see freedom from compulsive eating as something like this scripture. It's a way of ascending "the mountain of the Lord." It's a way of standing in his holy place, of being able to have a relationship with God. What that means is that if I'm going to continue eating responsibly and sensibly, if I'm going to keep from eating irresponsibly and compulsively, I have to keep "clean hands and a pure heart." I have to trust in and swear by the one true God rather than in the false idol of food.

It means that when I do something wrong, I need to own up to it, and if necessary make restitution or amends. It means that if there's something I'm holding onto that I need to eliminate from my life, I need to do that too. It means I'm responsible for examining myself to see if "if there be any wicked way in me" and asking God to "lead me in the way everlasting."

I can no longer just meander my way through life without thinking. I can't wake up each morning and just do what I feel like doing. Or eat what I feel like eating. Because I have a problem with compulsive eating, I have no choice but to practice diligence in this area. I also have another choice I need to make each day: to surrender my will and my food to God. To do and to eat the way he wants me to. It's not easy, but it can be done. I don't do it perfectly, but I'm learning every day.

Father, teach me to put you first and to walk in your ways. Amen.

by Debbie

May 23

Nothing is as wonderful as knowing Christ Jesus my Lord. I have given up everything else and count it all as garbage. All I want is Christ.
Philippians 3:8 CEV

Above all else, guard your heart, for everything you do flows from it.
Proverbs 4:23

I have this thing in my life. Some call it good and some call it ridiculous. I've always been a very organized person. I like everything in its place. Now, sometimes something ends up where it doesn't belong. Then I have to search all over for it. That makes me extremely frustrated, because—you know—everything has its place.

This makes me think about my mind and heart. Am I storing things in places that should not be there? Have those things become a disorganized mess?

When I think about my life, I can see that I'm storing fear in my heart. That's not where it belongs. Fear causes me to harbor thoughts of defeat. And really—does defeat belong in my mind?

Just as I would never put something metal in a microwave, I should be aware of what I'm storing in my mind and heart.

Father, please help me to store your word in my mind and heart. Help me to store only good and merciful things within me. Lord, keep everything within me organized according to your will. Help me live in integrity with what I choose to fill my mind. Help me live in integrity with the feelings I choose to harbor. Bless my thoughts and bless the feelings of my heart. I ask these things in the precious name of Jesus, amen.

by Nancy

May 24

What has been will be again, what has been done will be done again; there is nothing new under the sun.
Ecclesiastes 1:9

So I say, walk by the Spirit.
Galatians 5:16

As I write this, it is early 2021. We are still in the midst of the coronavirus pandemic, and our nation is divided along political extremes. It grieves my heart to see it so. Yet Americans have always had political differences. Religious differences. Racial differences. Since the founding of the United States, and before, when we were British colonies, and even before that when the land was populated only by its indigenous peoples.

In fact, competing ideologies and competing interests have been around since Cain and Abel. So, what we're experiencing, though it may be manifesting in unique ways in our time, isn't unique to the human experience.

How then should Christians respond? Jesus had some pretty strong words to say about loving our neighbor and brotherly love among believers. Paul exhorted us to walk by the Spirit. In other words, it's my job to sweep my side of the street (not someone else's). And to keep my ears open to how God is leading. Which means I may need to stop listening to and participating in a lot of the cultural noise going on in our media. Much of it is simply not my business. What is my business is to live the best life I can today, with God's help and with the strength he alone provides.

Lord, help me tune out the worst messages and listen to what you want from me. Let me always treat those around me as people of value. Amen.

by Debbie

May 25

Whoever desires to love life and see good days, let him keep his tongue from evil and his lips from speaking deceit.
1 Peter 3:10 ESV

Human beings were created in God's image. And when I gave my life to the Lord, I was filled with the Holy Spirit. When I accepted him into my heart, did I continue speaking evil against him? And because he is so good and pure, am I then being deceitful when I speak evil things about myself?

If I could only walk with the knowledge that God is right here. He's right here. He's within me. He is everything. He is beautiful. He is faithful. He is pure. He is strength.

If I really let that soak in deep, would it be easier to put those evil words aside? Would it be easier to say, "I'm sorry, Lord, for any mean or hateful words I've said about myself"?

Would I maybe see life in a different light?

I feel like the sun just might shine a little brighter in my world. I would see more good days instead of letting one little thing bring me down.

Our words have an impact on how we view ourselves and on our daily lives. God is telling us if we refrain from speaking evil and our lips from speaking deceit, we will love life and see good days.

Father, I value your word, so help me to walk in it. I believe your word, so help me to live by it. Help me to walk in the integrity of your word. That means that I choose to speak good and not evil, including about myself. In Jesus' name, amen.

by Nancy

May 26

Am I now trying to win the approval of human beings, or of God? Or am I trying to please people? If I were still trying to please people, I would not be a servant of Christ.
Galatians 1:10

I received an e-mail from a friend who is a missionary, along with her husband, overseas. Because of the real possibility of religious persecution there, including the threat of bodily harm, I can't say anything here that could identify them. She sends periodic updates to people who have agreed to pray for them and the success of their missions work. In the most recent one she talked about how God is uprooting and changing deep things in her, including "people-pleasing" and "approval-seeking."

Oh, how that convicted me. I'm so guilty of the same so much of the time. One example is a hobby, photography. I love it so much, not just because I love seeing and creating beautiful images, but because I love sharing them. I receive some approval for that. Another is being an instructor at a university. Am I there because it serves God, or because it brings me a certain status? That's something I need to pray about.

Yet there is purpose in everything. My friend also wrote: "Thanks be to God who has mercy to reveal these to us, so we may turn from them to him and his path. How I hurt my Master and his people when I follow my own agenda. And how my way of action does not bring the glory to him that he is due."

Father, reveal in me those things you want to remove from my life and my character, including the foods I'm holding onto that are holding me back from full obedience to you, your word, and your way. Please take them from me and replace them in my heart with a willingness to do your will. Amen.

by Debbie

May 27

He answered, "I heard you in the garden,
and I was afraid because I was naked; so I hid."
Genesis 3:10

I have more than a slight obsession with painting my house. It has been just about every color. My husband jokes that the walls are closing in on us; I just remind him that I'm insulating the house with all the layers. I do this for many reasons. First, one season I may like a certain color, then I get bored with it. Second, it makes my house feel fresh and clean. But mostly it's because I want my house to look nice at all times. I work hard to make that happen.

I wonder how many times I have put a "paint job" on myself. How many times have I tried to hide things from other people? How many times have I hidden the stains and the scratches in my life? Even tried to hide from God?

It's so easy to hide what I'm going through. It can be embarrassing to talk about. Sometimes I feel shame. But anyone can know the One who doesn't look at the paint but at the real self inside, and man does he love us! He loves us even with the stains and scratches. He wants us to come to him with no shame and no embarrassment. He loves us just the way we are! I want to strive for that place where I don't need to "paint" myself, where I can show people who I really am. And in God's eyes, each of us can truly claim to be special. To him.

Father, thank you for loving me no matter what and for never giving up on me. Help me become more "real" with those around me. Help me know that I'm a child of the King, that you're making the way straight for me, and that you're my deliverer and my friend. In Jesus' name, amen.

by Nancy

May 28

Instead, speaking the truth in love, we will grow to become in every respect the mature body of him who is the head, that is, Christ. From him the whole body, joined and held together by every supporting ligament, grows and builds itself up in love, as each part does its work.
Ephesians 4:15–16

One of the things I now understand is that compulsive overeating isolated me. I felt alone and different. Not as good. Not as attractive. It took extra effort to be social. When I was binging or doing my eating in secret, I didn't want to be around people. Having a lot of extra weight on my body made me want to "hide." I wore a lot of black clothes, because black is "slimming." That was another way of hiding the truth about myself.

Spending time with others who also struggle with weight and compulsive eating has helped a lot. I finally felt accepted. Not judged. And that was important. There will always be people who think they're better than I am, but that kind of arrogance is often hiding deep-seated feelings of inferiority that they're trying to hide; knowing that means I can feel sorry for someone like that.

If I want to be free of the shame that causes isolation, I need to let go of those things that cause them—I need to walk in integrity by sharing—even if it's just with one person—the worst part of me. By doing that, I realize that I'm the same as everyone else. We all fall short. We all have sinned. We all need God and each other. It's in finally being myself, in being who I really am before God, in being authentic, that I can finally let God change me. And I must change if I want to stop eating compulsively.

Father, make me aware of those things that make me want to hide from others and from you. Help me walk in authenticity and integrity. Amen.

by Debbie

May 29

Lying lips are an abomination to the Lord,
but those who act faithfully are his delight.
Proverbs 12:22

Now faith is confidence in what we hope for
and assurance about what we do not see.
Hebrews 11:1

I can't do it anymore. I'm at my wit's end. I work and work on it, and the scale doesn't budge. I don't want to do it anymore. I don't like exercising, so I won't do it anymore.

These are many of the things I have said to myself in a day of dieting. There are so many more lies that I've said to myself. Another "good one" is: *I may as well eat them all so they're not in the house anymore, and then I'll start fresh tomorrow.* How many tomorrows have come and gone and nothing has changed?

I need to tell myself that giving up is not an option. I need to take those two words—give up—out of my language. I need to constantly reaffirm the truth. Provide positive reinforcement to myself. Where do I get that reinforcement? God's word!

He tells us that in him we have the victory. Do you hear that? We HAVE the victory. The victory is not coming tomorrow. It's not coming next week. We have it right now. When I tell myself it's okay to give up, that's when failure comes in. Instead, I can press through each day. Yes, I might make a mistake. I might take an extra bite. Or grab some junk food. But as long as I don't give up, I have the victory. I'll just work a bit harder tomorrow. So whatever you do, tell yourself the truth. And DON'T GIVE UP!

Father, help me tell myself the truth, and give me the victory! Amen.

by Nancy

May 30

Then I heard another voice from heaven saying, "Come out of her, my people, lest you take part in her sins, lest you share in her plagues; for her sins are heaped high as heaven, and God has remembered her iniquities.
Revelation 18:4–5 ESV

Do not be unequally yoked with unbelievers. For what partnership has righteousness with lawlessness? Or what fellowship has light with darkness?
2 Corinthians 6:14 ESV

The idea of being set apart, of being "holy" is so unfamiliar in our culture. We're just everyday people going about our business, taking care of our families and our homes. Yet God has clearly called believers to be different. To be salt and light.

I've lived long enough to see how our culture has changed over the last fifty years or so. More change came during the 2020 COVID pandemic, not always for the greater good. I can see this most starkly in the field of entertainment. If I still had young children at home who might inadvertently turn to certain channels (or teens who might do so knowingly), I would get rid of cable and purchase only wholesome content (I still may do that). There are channels I rarely turn to, and when I occasionally do, I'm often shocked not by what I chose to watch, but by the content of the commercials. I shake my head and think: *Lord, help us all.*

God is also calling me to "come out of her" in the way that I eat. He wants me to be holy in *everything*, including with my food. He wants me to be pure in mind, body, and actions. I'm part of the church that he is making ready, as a bride for her bridegroom.

Father, remind me how important it is to be holy in everything, whether it's what I put in my mind or what I physically put into my body. Amen.

by Debbie

May 31

"Not everyone who says to me, 'Lord, Lord,' will enter the kingdom of heaven, but only the one who does the will of my Father who is in heaven."
Matthew 7:21

Today's evangelical Christians tend to focus on the positive aspects of God's character: his love, comfort, salvation, and how he provides hope, provision, and purpose. But there are some hard truths in the Bible too. God is also holy, just, and pure. And here, Jesus doesn't mince words. I don't believe this means that Christians have to be (or even can be) perfect. But God does want my obedience. He wants me to seek to do his will to the best of my ability. Or it might be better to say to the best of the ability and strength he gives me.

I fall short frequently. And yet I'm learning. Every day I learn a little more—if I pay attention. The hard part is when I examine my own heart. I discover that I feel like Isaiah the prophet who said, "Woe to me! . . . I am ruined! For I am a man of unclean lips, and I live among a people of unclean lips, and my eyes have seen the King, the Lord Almighty." The more I study, the more I realize both how little I know and how imperfect I am.

The good news is that God knows this about me and loves me anyway. And he has made a way for all my sins to be covered and cleansed—through Jesus' death on the cross.

At the same time, he still wants my allegiance, my obedience, and my desire to do his will, including with how I eat. To do that I have to study his word, and I must stay in touch with him daily.

Father, help me at those instances when I recognize the depths of my sin and disobedience. Cleanse me from all unrighteousness and give me the knowledge of your will and the strength to carry it out. In Jesus' name, amen.

by Debbie

WILLINGNESS

We must become truly willing to change.

Cry of Our Hearts

June 1

Commit your way to the Lord; trust in him, and he will act.
Psalm 37:5

"If anyone wants to come after Me, he must deny himself, take up his cross, and follow Me."
Mark 8:34 NASB

When it comes to weight loss, for people who are true over-eaters, for people who are obese and have never been able to overcome it, our society tells the worst lie there is: That if we want to lose weight, we just need enough willpower.

The truth is that willpower is the exact *opposite* of what we need. The idea behind willpower is not just strength of will, but it implies self-will. And it is self-will that has put us in this predicament. In my case, it was self-will run riot. I wanted to eat whatever I wanted, whenever I wanted. And not have to suffer the consequences. When I first heard this truth, it seemed counterintuitive. I had heard my whole life that I just needed willpower. I just needed self-discipline. When I heard that it was *willingness* rather than willpower that I needed, it took me a long time to comprehend the concept. What was this **willingness**?

I discovered that it means I become willing to do things God's way and not my way. I recognize that if I disagree with God, guess who's wrong? It meant being willing to give up my way and try things God's way, even when it comes to food.

I don't do it perfectly, but I return to willingness whenever I mess up and whenever I feel stuck. Becoming willing to do things God's way hasn't let me down yet.

Father, make me willing today. Let your will, not mine be done. Amen.

by Debbie

June 2

For we know that our old self was crucified with him so that the body ruled by sin might be done away with, that we should no longer be slaves to sin.
Romans 6:6

When I first started this weight-loss journey, it never occurred to me to give my food to God. It was something I had control over, and I liked having that control. I liked eating what I wanted when I wanted.

But as with anything that's addictive, control is an illusion. Eventually, what you want to control—because you like the feeling it gives you—controls you instead. You become enslaved to it.

So I asked the Lord what he wanted me to give up. And then I asked him, and continue to ask him every morning, to give me the strength to do it. If he wants me to do this, then he's going to have to help me, because I couldn't even take the first step on my own power.

I even had to pray to be willing, and after a few times of praying that, I was suddenly given the willingness. It appeared, as if by magic. And as long as I'm willing to do what God wants me to do, as long as I continue to ask him for help, somehow I can do it. That's the miracle I've experienced.

And I really like feeling lighter, in body and spirit, even though I still have more to go on this journey. I can see the difference, as can others, and I'm looking forward to losing even more. That is more rewarding to me than anything I could eat. It feels better than anything will ever taste.

Jesus, Lord of my life, please keep me willing to do your will. Then show me what you want me to do. Then help me to do it. Amen.

by Debbie

June 3

But the Helper, the Holy Spirit, whom the Father will send in my name, he will teach you all things and bring to your remembrance all that I have said.
John 14:26 ESV

How many times have I had a part-time relationship with the Father? You know, the kind where I only go to him when I need something or to say a quick thank you.

I need to have daily personal fellowship with my King. I need to get that daily bread into my life. If I fill up on his bread, then I won't need the other bread quite so much. He wants to be my King, my Savior, my Healer, my Friend. He longs to be in complete fellowship at all times with each of us.

So, as I walk this weight-loss journey, if I include him in more of my decisions, just maybe I can see more favorable results. Like for breakfast, I could stand at the refrigerator and ask, "Lord, what should I have today?" When I want to grab a treat, "Lord, should I have this?" The true test will come when I hear his answer and then follow it.

Some days I still make the wrong choice. But if I turn to him every day, each time I want to eat something, it will get easier to obey him. It will get easier to hear his answer, and easier not to be defiant. I know he will bless me each time I choose to listen and obey. He longs to be my Savior in this area of my life too. He longs to be my hero. He longs to be the Helper who will get me all the way through to my goal weight. Will I allow him to be those things to me?

Father, make me willing to be open to you. Make me willing to turn to you instead of to the food. Make me willing to seek you out every day. Amen.

by Nancy

June 4

Jesus replied, "Very truly I tell you, no one can see the kingdom of God unless they are born again.
John 3:3

Do not conform to the pattern of this world, but be transformed by the renewing of your mind. Then you will be able to test and approve what God's will is—his good, pleasing and perfect will.
Romans 12:2

One of the things that Jesus did for us on the cross is to make a way for us to receive the spirit of God into our lives—into our very beings. It's what the Bible refers to as being "born again" in John's gospel. Without that experience, we can't even truly start the transformation process that will help us live the way God intended. And what is that process? It's how God begins to remove the defects in our character, those things that cause us to act in ways that are contrary to God's will for us.

Of course, one of the ways I acted contrary to God's will was to eat compulsively. God's will for me has always been for me to maintain a healthy body weight. But I couldn't do that, because I used food as a way to comfort myself, as a way not to have to feel certain feelings. And that made food into an idol in my life. I just didn't have the strength to overcome my compulsion on my own. I still don't. But Jesus does.

Father, there are times I've been hurt and times I've been fearful. I've been unwise and insensitive. Remove these defects of character. Help me to have faith and be bold, to love despite hurt and betrayal, and most of all to think the way you want me to think and act the way you want me to act. Transform my heart and mind. Make me more like you. In Jesus' name, amen.

by Debbie

June 5

Therefore, brothers and sisters, we have an obligation—but it is not to the flesh, to live according to it. For if you live according to the flesh, you will die; but if by the Spirit you put to death the misdeeds of the body, you will live.
Romans 8:12–13

"Being obedient to God does not always guarantee that He will make the path easy. It is my role as His child. Sometimes, God leads us to do things that are seemingly impossible. However, His call is simply to be obedient, to be a willing vessel. He will take care of the rest!" — Steve Cleary, CEO/Founder, RevelationMedia.

The interesting thing about Steve Cleary is that he had a speech impediment, yet God called him to a public role in his ministry in which he would need to speak in front of people and to the media. He was reluctant, but finally obedient, and in time God took away his speech impediment.

It's like that when I'm attempting to be obedient to God with my food. I may need to suffer through the hunger pangs (real or emotional) that result from learning to say no to myself, learning not to give in to what I want in the moment. Learning to be obedient to God rather than to my flesh.

Obedience is hard. Saying no to the flesh is difficult. And yet we're called to do it anyway. If I don't, the consequences are dire. If I continue in my self-indulgence, I will die much earlier than I'm meant to.

Father, you said that I was crucified with Christ, that he lives in me. You said that you would give me the power to overcome. Yet my flesh continues to contend with my spirit; I need your help in my weakness. In Jesus' name, amen.

by Debbie

June 6

Create in me a clean heart, God, and renew a steadfast spirit within me. Do not cast me away from Your presence, and do not take Your Holy Spirit from me. Restore to me the joy of Your salvation and sustain me with a willing spirit. Lord, open my lips, so that my mouth may declare Your praise. For You do not delight in sacrifice, otherwise I would give it; You do not take pleasure in burnt offering. The sacrifices of God are a broken spirit; A broken and a contrite heart, God, You will not despise.
Psalm 51:10–12, 15–17 NASB

"Please wash me anew in the wine of Your blood." That's a line in a song that I like. It's talking about becoming new. About renewing our faith. My prayer is that my faith never gets old.

I find that if I would only search out God every day, he has something new to teach me. He has so much joy to share with me. I'm awed about his love for me.

But on some days, I'm a jerk. I know this. And if you say you're not, then you're not being honest. We all have things in our lives that we need to work on.

We all have things where God clears his throat and says, "What were you thinking?" It could be that you judge people. It could be that you gossip. It could be that you let small things your family does irritate you instead of letting them go.

Oh God, create in me a clean heart. Don't let me act "holier than thou." Lord, give me a willing spirit. I just want to follow you. I want to walk right behind you and beside you. Lord, I want to love you with my whole heart. I want to be pure in heart. God, I just want you. I just want to be in your presence. Oh God, I long to be in your presence. I love you, Lord, with everything within me. Oh God, forgive me and wash me anew. In Jesus' name, amen.

by Nancy

June 7

Therefore, if anyone is in Christ, he is a new creation.
The old has passed away; behold, the new has come.
2 Corinthians 5:17

When I first became willing to face my weight problem head on, I had to ask myself: "Am I really willing to change?" Change the way I think, the way I act, the way I eat? Change patterns of behavior that I have been entrenched for years?

I had to come to a point where I was willing to say, "God, I've been really stupid. Look at me. I don't have to tell you that. I've been a fool. I've messed up my life entirely. I have no wisdom of my own. Please show me what to do. I'm willing to do whatever you want me to do to overcome this problem."

That was the starting point. Being willing. Then I really had to listen and do the things God was showing me, either by whispering things to my spirit, in what I was reading, or in what I heard from others. I went to a twelve-step meeting. I listened. I tried some of the things I heard people talk about, like giving up refined sugar. Like measuring my portions. Like finding others with more experience who gave me good advice.

But that was just a beginning. What I have discovered since then is that I have to pray for willingness daily. I have to surrender daily. Especially when it comes to food. But in other things in my life as well. When I find that I'm stuck, when I'm struggling, it almost invariably comes down to self-will. That is, me having too much of it and me not having enough willingness to do what God wants.

Father, you know that I am full of self-will in my rebellious little heart. Please give me a heart that seeks your will instead. In Jesus' name, amen.

by Debbie

June 8

Since most of our problems—and all of our bad habits—didn't develop overnight, it's unrealistic to expect them to go away immediately. Contrary to popular book titles, there are no Easy Steps to Maturity *or* Secrets of Instant Sainthood.
Rick Warren in The Purpose Driven Life

One catch phrase I've heard often is that the journey to long-term recovery from eating compulsively is "simple, but not easy." The hard truth is that it takes focus and work, and you must become willing to do what it takes to achieve it.

At first all I could do was pray for willingness, because my rebellious heart certainly was not willing to change, nor was I willing to do the work. I wanted to continue eating what I loved whenever I wanted to eat it. There were things I was sure I could never give up. I was skeptical that it was even possible. After all, the statistics for long-term weight loss are miserable.

I finally became willing to do whatever it takes, but not until after weeks of praying for willingness. Just short, quick prayers, said frequently throughout those weeks: "Lord, please help me to be willing, because I'm not." And then one day I was.

Apparently—who knew?—when you pray for something, sometimes the Lord answers yes. I'm being facetious, of course, because it should be obvious that when we pray according to God's will that he will give us what we ask for. And it is God's will that we live victoriously in him. It's how we live in a way that lets others know that it's truly possible for our bodies to be a living witness to God's power and, more importantly, his love.

Father, make me willing to do what I am often at first unwilling to do. Help me to continue this journey to better health, one day at a time. Amen.

by Debbie

June 9

If you are willing and obedient, you will eat the good things of the land.
Isaiah 1:19

As I write today, it is Easter. I have thought a lot about what happened to our Lord that week. All the torture he went through. All the pain he endured. What he had to give up for us.

I wonder why, knowing all that, it's so hard for me to give up simple things? He was willing to give it all for me. Yet I'm unwilling to give it all to him. I'm unwilling to say I won't buy anymore candy or soda pop. Those things that are only harming my body.

It comes down to being willing. I've heard people use the description "strong-willed child." I think about what that really means. In my life being strong-willed is NOT good. Not when I'm harming my body. If I'm going to be strong-willed, then I want it to be toward the Lord. I want to be strong-willed enough to eat as he wants me to eat. I want to be strong-willed in walking the healthy path that he desires for me. Is that submission? Submitting to the Lord and choosing to do what is right?

The Lord has been talking to me about behaviors lately. I'll be diving into that and seeing what else he wants to show me. But the first step is to work on not being so strong-willed. Giving my life and my food—all of it—over to him. Giving up the things I know are harming me.

Father, please help me to walk in the ways that you have designed so that I would be healthy and full of joy. Lord, please help me to work on my willingness to make right decisions. Good decisions. Thank you, Lord, for all that you were willing to do for me. May I be able give a portion back to you. In Jesus' name, amen.

by Nancy

June 10

If you fully obey the Lord your God and carefully follow all his commands I give you today, the Lord your God will set you high above all the nations on earth. All these blessings will come on you and accompany you if you obey the Lord your God.
Deuteronomy 28:1–2

I've been thinking a lot lately about what I put in my mouth. About how many times I put things in my mouth. I could blame fibromyalgia. Fibro makes it really difficult to exercise. But it should not stop me from eating healthier. In fact, healthier eating might help. I could also blame my medications, I'm not discounting them. Some meds contribute to weight gain, but not mine. So I can take that excuse out. It's so hard to look in the mirror and realize that I'm responsible for my weight problem.

The truth is that I haven't wanted to take full responsibility. I haven't been willing. And that has "given" me the out to eat how I want. I know I need to cut out snacking. I don't need to be putting things in my mouth all night long. I need to find better habits to replace that urge to want to eat all the time. I also need to take the time to figure out what healthy meals look like. I don't like to cook, so it's easy to just whip up a hotdish. Or throw a pizza in the oven. I've trained myself to an unhealthy way of cooking; now I need to take the time to train myself to a healthy way of cooking. That means that I need to be diligent about it. I need to take responsibility for what I've done and be willing to change it now.

Lord, I repent for all that I have done to contribute to my weight gain and for ignoring how I'm eating compulsively. Please bless me in building new healthy habits that are pleasing to you. Make me willing. In Jesus' name, amen.

by Nancy

June 11

You need to persevere so that when you have done the will of God, you will receive what he has promised.
Hebrews 10:36

Our Father in heaven, hallowed be your name, your kingdom come, your will be done, on earth as it is in heaven.
Matthew 6:9–10

The reasons why you overeat will come to you. And even if they don't (not everything has come to me yet), what matters is taking action. I didn't choose to be abstinent from sugar until I started going to twelve-step meetings, and even then it took me a few weeks before I decided to become accountable to at least one other person, after which I finally stopped eating sugar. But that was just the first step. The compulsion to overeat is about much more than the food. What and how much I eat is just the tip of the iceberg. I had to *work* at it, which involved ongoing self-reflection and a lot of writing. Going to one twelve-step meeting a week keeps me accountable. And there are other things I do every day. I read relevant literature, study the Bible, pray, and keep track of my food using an app.

To lose more weight, though, I need to pay closer attention to my current diet, and I must become willing to make additional changes. I haven't been willing yet. So I'm praying for willingness.

Sometimes that's how you start. You're not willing, so you ask God to make you willing. And then one day you're willing, because that's a prayer God never says no to. To be willing to do his will? Does God ever say no to that?!

Father, please make me willing to do what you want me to do today. In Jesus' name, amen.

by Debbie

June 12

And I am sure of this, that he who began a good work in you will bring it to completion at the day of Jesus Christ.
Philippians 1:6 ESV

Change can be a good thing, right? I wonder what would happen if I took steps each day to change. If I take a "baby step" each day, just maybe I'll start seeing change in my life.

Maybe today just one time instead of grabbing a cookie, try eating a banana. Then maybe by the end of the week, I'll have chosen quite a few bananas and zero cookies.

For most of us—for me, certainly—change has to come gradually. I tend to gravitate toward fad diets and try to change too fast. Some of those diets have good ideas, but they're still too much too fast for me to handle.

I think of things that I have had to work through with the Lord over my lifetime. And I can see where he took things one at a time. He didn't one day wake me up and say, "Today we're dealing with all the junk in your life." He took things slowly, and when I look back I can say I've grown. If he had done it all at once, would I be where I am today? Or would it have been too frustrating, causing me to give up?

I'd much rather lose all the weight NOW. Of course that's not going to happen. But I can start with ten minutes on the treadmill, and maybe tomorrow I'll do fifteen. Today, I can change just one thing. Why not lose it at a pace that means it won't come back? I can take it one step, one success at a time.

Father, make me willing to take the first step. And then tomorrow I can take another. In Jesus' name, amen.

by Nancy

June 13

The Lord makes firm the steps of the one who delights in him.
Psalm 37:23

At some point in any weight-loss effort, you reach a plateau, and yet you feel you need to lose more. When this happened to me, God showed me that it was part of the journey. I needed time to get used to my new way of eating and used to a smaller body size.

When this happened, I also needed to trust God. He's the one in charge of my goal weight, not me. And I realized that this plateau was also part of his plan for me. I needed time to adjust. Time to get used to new habits. Time for my thinking and feelings to catch up. It was so wonderful feeling lighter and smaller; I needed some time to start feeling heavy again.

And that is beginning to happen. I still need to continue on this journey and lose that heaviness. I have to continue to pray for the willingness to make more changes, to continue to surrender every day.

For me, this journey has been for the long haul. I lost weight slowly and did so intentionally. I knew that if I ate more during the weight-loss period, if I ate at the calorie level expected to maintain a healthy weight, that I would be more likely to keep the weight off. And so far it has worked. And when the right time comes, all in God's plan and timing, I'll be willing and able to take the next steps.

Father, thank you for teaching me what I need to know at the moment I need to know it. Make me willing to wait when I need to wait, move when I need to move, and change when you want me to change. In Jesus' name, amen.

by Debbie

June 14

You have searched me, Lord, and you know me. You know when I sit and when I rise; you perceive my thoughts from afar. You discern my going out and my lying down; you are familiar with all my ways.
Psalm 139:1–3

If I believe the Bible, and I do, I see that God knows me better than I know myself. He not only knows my personality and my innermost being, but he knows my body, how it works, my habits, and my weaknesses and strengths with food.

Therefore, why shouldn't I ask God to show me what to eat, how to eat, and when to eat? I should! Over time, God has shown me what I need to abstain from, what tools to use to keep me on "the straight and narrow," and what specifically works and doesn't work for me in my diet.

I heard one person say she can't eat any kind of nuts, because they make her nutty! That's a humorous way of looking at a truth about her. But I've found that I have very specific trouble spots. I can eat low-salt almonds sensibly, a small handful at a time. But I can't buy cashews anymore—I'll scarf them. And keep scarfing them until I've blown my calorie allotment for the day. I can do the same with corn chips. I can measure out a specific amount and not reach for more. But that's not true of potato chips—there's something about them that's so addictive that I've had to put them on my "dangerous foods" list.

Have I ever gone back to trying to eat cashews? Yes, and every time I have learned the same lesson over again: God knows best, and I should listen and obey him.

Father, show me what and how you want me to eat and then help me be willing to follow what you have shown me. In Jesus' name, amen.

by Debbie

June 15

Set your minds on things that are above, not on things that are on earth.
Colossians 3:2 ESV

"Father, if you are willing, take this cup from me;
yet not my will, but yours be done."
Luke 22:42

How many times have I asked the Lord to take this food addiction/weight problem from me? How many times have I tried fad diets? I've tried many, and I have begged God to please just take this cup from me.

I know I don't have the willpower to do it. None of us do. But I know Someone who can help me. He can teach me, and I can learn along the way how to walk a better walk in this journey of life. I need to learn that for all areas of my life.

He wants to teach me that my own willpower is useless, but I can become willing to be obedient to him. I can become willing to do what he asks me to do to lose the weight. To overcome the addiction. He also wants to teach me patience. We have become a society of "I want it now." And with that attitude comes greed and selfishness. Those are attributes he doesn't want me to have. Yet if I keep relying on him and give him my attention, I'll finally learn what he wants to teach me. If I stay willing, how much better off I'll be in so many areas of my life.

Father, please help me to set my mind on you. Lord, I need to become less about trying to get what I want and more about finding out what you want. Your ways are better than anything I could ask or imagine. Your ways bring life and love. Please open my ears and eyes to hear and see what you have for me! In Jesus' name, amen.

by Nancy

June 16

Do your own work well, and then you will have something to be proud of. But don't compare yourself with others. We each must carry our own load.
Galatians 6:4–5 CEV

Though I have lost fifty pounds in the last two years, I still have more to lose to attain a truly healthy body weight. I'm certainly not "skinny" (though I don't ever expect to be—just healthy). I've given myself a while to adjust to the change, and now it's time to see what else God wants me to do, what other changes he wants me to make so I can move forward.

To do that, I have to take responsibility for myself, my body, and my actions. I must take responsibility for my decisions. It may be true that my body retains weight more easily than others. It may be true that I didn't learn good eating habits as a child. That doesn't absolve me of the responsibility to learn new habits and take those direct actions that are needed to accomplish what God wants me to do.

It's time for some self-examination: Is there an area in my life or in my eating where I'm still being rebellious? Is there a habit I'm clinging to that the Lord wants me to let go? Am I spending too much time doing one thing when the Lord wants me to spend that time learning how to eat better, how to cook healthier foods? Am I willing to examine an entirely new way of eating at the Lord's direction? I am.

Father, if I'm not willing, please make me willing. When I am *willing, please show me what you want me to do so that I'll know it without question. When I'm weak, give me the strength to follow through with your will for my life. In Jesus' name, amen.*

by Debbie

June 17

Trust in the Lord with all your heart and lean not on your own understanding; in all your ways submit to him, and he will make your paths straight.
Proverbs 3:5–6

One of the hardest lessons for me to learn in this weight-loss journey has been to "let go." Why do I so often want to hold onto things so tightly? Why am I so afraid of change? Of giving up something that has worked in one way and hurt me in another?

Yet it's only in the act of letting go that I become free. There is an illustration of this in John Bunyan's *The Pilgrim's Progress* as the main character, Christian, comes to belief in Christ and his heavy burden is lifted. He lets it go. Another comes from the book *Drop the Rock*, in which there's a description of the following scenario: A group takes off in a boat and suddenly they see someone jump into the water after them, hoping to catch the boat. But the person starts to sink, because she's carrying a huge rock that's weighing her down. The people in the boat shout, "Drop the rock!" And it's only when she does that she can swim freely and catch up with the boat and be pulled aboard to safety.

In my case, I'm often willfully holding onto some sin or other, and then God tells me, "It's time to let go of that." Recently it was a set of romance novels stored on my Kindle. It was time to delete them. Most often, it's some food or another that's a problem for me. It might be a favorite that I really don't want to give up. But if I want true freedom, true safety, and true healing, I need to do what God asks. I need to let it go.

Father, show me what you want me to let go, and give me the power to do it so I can walk in your way and your wisdom. In Jesus name, amen.

by Debbie

June 18

For he was saying to him, come out of the man, you unclean spirit.
Mark 5:8 ESV

What am I slave to? What is holding me back? What is controlling my life? I know that I'm a slave to fear. I'm a slave to food. I'm a slave to soda pop. Anything that I fight to get out of my life—yet still controls me—is something I'm a slave to.

I sometimes fear what will happen if I lose weight. Will I change? Will my marriage change? Who will I be without the fat? Fear controls so many areas of my life. I'm afraid to go out and meet new people, afraid to let loose and just be myself.

I'm so glad that I serve a God who will help me break those bonds. He will set me free. He *has* set the captive free. That includes me. If only I would hold my hands out and let him cut off the chains. What's holding me back? What's stopping me from allowing God to set me free from fear? Free from obesity? Free from pain and sadness? I'm the only one holding myself back.

I heard a saying the other day that all things can be mended. Not with time, but with intention. I need to be intent on wanting to change. I need to be intent on letting God cut me free. My focus needs to be on what there is to gain from change instead of what I may have to give up. What will I gain? Happiness, peace, health, joy. The list could go on and on. There's so much more to gain than there is by continuing to live in bondage.

Father, break my chains. I repent for allowing spirits to control my every move and ask that you would set me free. Break me free from the things that enslave me. I long for freedom. I long for peace. I long to live a long, healthy life. Make me willing to change and follow your way. In Jesus' name, amen.

by Nancy

June 19

Go, my people, enter your rooms and shut the doors behind you; hide yourselves for a little while until his wrath has passed by.
Isaiah 26:20

Here I am! I stand at the door and knock. If anyone hears my voice and opens the door, I will come in and eat with that person, and they with me.
Revelation 3:20

I like the imagery of a door. It's an entryway and an exit. It can be open or shut. You're either inside or out. This weight-loss journey has been like opening and walking through a door. Have I closed the door behind me to the past? I've certainly closed the door to some things. I've closed the door on refined sugar. I've closed the door on binging.

I've also opened the door to many things. To a closer and more trusting relationship with God. I've opened the door wider so that I can take a few steps closer to freedom from many of my fears, which is what happens when you begin to trust God more.

If I'm inside, a closed door protects me from what's going on outside. During Passover, the blood splashed on the lintels and posts of closed doors protected the Israelites from the death of their firstborn. If I'm outside and there's someone I want to see who's inside, I'm prevented from fellowshipping with that person unless I have permission to enter. If I'm inside and someone knocks, I have to open the door to let the person in.

With this weight-loss journey, it's God who has opened the door for me. Because of that, I've been willing to cross the threshold and enter a whole new world. A much better one.

Father, thank you for opening the door for me and letting me in. Amen.

by Debbie

June 20

Indeed, if we consider the unblushing promises of reward and the staggering nature of the rewards promised in the Gospels, it would seem that Our Lord finds our desires, not too strong, but too weak. We are half-hearted creatures, fooling about with drink and sex and ambition when infinite joy is offered us, like an ignorant child who wants to go on making mud pies in a slum because he cannot imagine what is meant by the offer of a holiday at the sea. We are far too easily pleased.
C. S. Lewis in The Weight of Glory

No mere man has ever seen, heard, or even imagined what wonderful things God has ready for those who love the Lord.
1 Corinthians 2:9

I was a little girl making mud pies in the slum. At first I was completely oblivious to the idea that God wanted to help me with my eating problem or that he was waiting for me to ask before he helped me. When I realized that he was willing, I wasn't. I held onto the food as a system of self-comfort for so long that I didn't know how to or if I could let go. And I didn't really want to.

I mean, how can a person not ever eat sugar again? How could I possibly enjoy life without the foods I liked to eat? How could I eat differently from the rest of my family, who could continue to eat things I no longer could? Would I be relegated to eating celery and carrots for the rest of my life?

The good news is that when I finally was willing to leave the mud pies and follow my Father's will for me, it wasn't more than I could handle. And though sometimes it hasn't been easy, the rewards far outstrip the difficulties.

Father, thank you for leading me to a holiday at the sea. Amen.

by Debbie

June 21

There is a time for everything, and a season for every activity under the heavens.
Ecclesiastes 3:1

I used to smoke. I really wanted to quit but couldn't seem to do it. Then one day it clicked. I read scripture when I needed a cigarette. The habit just faded away. I knew smoking wasn't pleasing to God, so I thought he'd want me to quit immediately, but there was a timing to it that he knew meant I would succeed.

How many times have I tried diets that just don't "take"? I get frustrated and give up. Then I think, okay, this is it! I'm going to try again! And—wham!—it happens again. I fail and give up.

I realized that I have to take the time to talk to God about the timing of it all. Are there other things happening that may hinder my success at this moment? That's not to say "do your own thing." But I need to find a balance where I can make smaller, healthier choices. That may be what gives me the ability to achieve lifelong success.

God knows when that moment will come. That moment I'll know that I know—this is it. There will be a lifelong change. A whole change of heart. Wanting to be healthy. Wanting to get the weight off. Wanting to turn an addiction into a closer relationship with God.

I once heard a pastor say that when you repent of something, picture a hole in your body where you removed the bad habit. He said make sure you fill the hole with something good. It's up to me to fill that hole. Fill it with journaling. Or with reading God's word. Or fill it with time with the Lord.

Father, help me listen to you and follow your timing in all areas of my life. Fill each hole with something better, something good and healthy. In Jesus' name, amen.

by Nancy

June 22

I have been crucified with Christ; and it is no longer I who live, but Christ lives in me; and the life which I now live in the flesh I live by faith in the Son of God, who loved me and gave Himself up for me.
Galatians 2:20 NASB

Funny how after you start eating healthy things, the unhealthy ones feel like a lump of lead in your tummy. A friend once described donuts as "grease and sugar." Nobody would eat a pile of grease just because it was mixed with sugar, but in the past that's exactly what I put in my body. Ugh. Now it seems like poison.

So, what is it that will keep me from making those bad choices again? Is it the fear of dying young? The fear of becoming disabled by disease (due to obesity) as I get older?

Those fears alone will not keep me going. As my body gets smaller, those things will no longer be the great threat that they were. No, the only thing that will keep me going on this weight-loss journey is a willingness to obey God. As the other motivations fade, only the desire to please Jesus will sustain me. Otherwise, I risk complacency and falling into even greater sin.

I'm reminded of what happened to King David. After being hunted by King Saul, he was probably saying to himself, "I've been through hell and back again. I deserve a little ME time. Let the other men go to war. I'll stay home and relax and enjoy myself." That choice led to his affair with Bathsheba and to his decision to murder her husband to cover up an unplanned pregnancy. An entire family, an entire *nation* suffered the consequences.

Let that not happen to me, Lord. Let me be diligent, and when I need to rest, may it be at your will rather than my own. When I have no strength, help me, Lord, to trust in you. Let my greatest desire be to please you. Amen.

by Debbie

June 23

Our mouths were filled with laughter, our tongues with songs of joy. Then it was said among the nations, "The Lord has done great things for them." The Lord has done great things for us, and we are filled with joy.
Psalm 126:2–3

At the time of this writing, I have lost fifty pounds with God's help, and I have kept it off for almost two years. My job has been to ask God to help me see the truth and for willingness and help along the way, and he has been faithful to answer those ongoing prayers.

At one point I felt God nudge me to give up artificial sweeteners, especially sugar-free mints, which had helped me early on when I first gave up sugar. After making that change, I had a low-grade headache for a week, which shows me it's likely that my system was ridding itself of the unnatural chemicals in the artificial sweeteners.

I've also continued to ask God to show me what changes he wants me to make in my life. That has included asking God to remove those defects in my character that keep me from living according to his purpose for me. From one of the devotionals I read daily I have learned that it is being in denial, an inflated ego, and self-will that will always lead me down the path into enslavement to and self-destruction with food. So I must pray to be free of those things. And God is always working to free me, because he is faithful. The Bible reminds me that I should "bless the Lord and not forget the glorious things he does for me" (*The Living Bible*).

Father, help me to remember all the wonderful things you have done for me in my life and in the life of each person I love. And thank you for the things you are planning to bless me with in the future. In Jesus' name, amen.

by Debbie

June 24

So then, just as you received Christ Jesus as Lord, continue to live your lives in him, rooted and built up in him, strengthened in the faith as you were taught and overflowing with thankfulness.
Colossians 2:6–7

Today I was driving and looking at all the fields that have been planted. I could see little sprouts sticking out of the ground. I was thinking about how the farmer tilled that land. He then put the seed in the dirt. The dirt took that seed and helped it grow.

I have some things in my past that were full of dirt. Yet during those times God was planting little seeds to help me grow from those experiences. From those places in my life, I can choose to grow, or I can choose to wither up and die. The Lord has done what he needs to do. He planted seeds in the midst of the chaos. The seeds might have been praying family or friends. Gentle words I didn't realize were from him. Or maybe he spoke very clearly. It all boils down to whether I take the seeds and let them grow or reject them and refuse to make any progress.

For most of my life he has planted seeds, and I have listened and then turned away. But there's still time for me, and there's still time for you. We can choose to take the seeds and grow. Grow in knowledge of how to be healthy. Grow in knowledge of just how much he loves us and only wants the best for us. It's time to nurture the seedlings so they can flourish and grow.

Father, help me to see the seeds planted in my life. The seeds that you have planted to help me live a safe, healthy, joyful, and peaceful life. Help me choose to grab hold of the seeds and grow. Grow mighty and strong. Thank you for caring so much for me that you took the time to plant those seeds. In Jesus' name, amen.

by Nancy

June 25

The world and its desires pass away,
but whoever does the will of God lives forever.
1 John 2:17

God is powerful and yet interested in everything about me. He wants me to succeed, to win the race, to carry out the Great Commission, to help others, to lose the weight. He will give me what I need to accomplish his will in my life. If I ask him. And if I'm willing to do what he asks.

That's the tough part, isn't it? What if he asks me to pray more? To read scripture more? To give up my favorite foods? To weigh and measure what I eat? Am I willing to take the actions he wants me to take?

If Jesus stood in front of me right now and asked me to complete a task, wouldn't I do that right away if it were in my power? And what if it didn't seem to be in my power? Would I step out in faith, trusting that he would provide whatever means and abilities I needed in order to accomplish what he asked me to do?

That's the meaning of calling him Lord. Of calling him my King. I think of the lyrics to a favorite song:

Amazing love, how can it be?
That You, my King would die for me.

Jesus is standing in front of you right now, asking you to do his will. If you're not willing to do it, you can pray to be willing. And you can step out in faith and take the action he's asking of you.

Father, help me to be willing to do your will every day. Amen.

by Debbie

June 26

Then the Lord said to Cain, "Why are you angry? Why is your face downcast? If you do what is right, will you not be accepted? But if you do not do what is right, sin is crouching at your door; it desires to have you, but you must rule over it."
Genesis 4:6

I can take one of two paths. They are set before me every day. The path that leads to destruction or the path that leads to life. When Cain was confronted with this choice, it led to the death of his brother, Abel, to banishment, to a bad name, and a host of other awful consequences.

Every day, sin is crouching at my door, desiring to have me, and I have the choice whether to rule over it. What I have discovered is that the choice isn't about willpower, about rigidly relying on my *own* power. It *is* about choosing not to give in to self-will. It's about trusting God, even when things don't always make sense. It's about being willing to allow God to work in me and in my life in ways that I don't always understand.

I used to think that God was being mean to Cain. After all, God rejected Cain's offering. We don't know exactly why God did that—maybe Cain hadn't given God the best of what he had. Maybe he had scrimped, not given enough. Maybe it was his attitude. But God did give Cain a chance to make it right; instead, Cain gave in to hurt feelings and jealousy, which led to anger, which led to murder, which led to everything that followed.

My choices are the same with food. I can give in to my feelings or I can ask God to help me. That's my choice every day.

Father, remind me every day that I must rely on you, your power, and your strength to get me through my worst temptations. In Jesus' name, amen.

by Debbie

June 27

It is for freedom that Christ has set us free. Stand firm, then, and do not let yourselves be burdened again by a yoke of slavery.
Galatians 5:1

I used to have this thing where I would hit myself. I know it sounds ridiculous. I grew out of that phase, but I have realized that I still abuse myself. I just picked a different form of abuse.

We all know the problems that come with overeating. We all know the results of obesity, the health risks. We may even have seen family or friends die from those results. So if we know all that, then we can call it what it is—self-abuse. So then the question becomes: Why do we abuse ourselves?

It could come from different causes. Some things we may know right away. Some things we may need to have the Lord reveal to us, and I believe if we ask, he'll show us. So then the question becomes: Do we want to know? Sometimes there are issues we would rather leave buried in the past. I'm all for that if it's been dealt with and healed. If not, you can see what it's doing to your health and body by letting it fester.

We need to evaluate whether we've dealt with the past and if we've forgiven where forgiveness is needed. Have you forgiven yourself? I find it much easier to forgive someone else than I do myself. I tend to judge myself quite harshly, so I need to walk daily in forgiving myself. That can be a tough one, but God is faithful. If we ask.

Father, reveal to me the truth about myself. Help me to see what I'm doing to my body, and why. Then show me what I need to do to walk in your way instead of my way. To accept your healing and move on into your freedom. In Jesus' name, amen.

by Nancy

June 28

Heal me, Lord, and I will be healed;
save me and I will be saved, for you are the one I praise.
Jeremiah 17:14

Sometimes God heals instantly. Sometimes he uses the people around us to heal (such as the doctors and nurses who treat us when we're ill or have had an accident), and sometimes he takes the long way 'round. I think that's because often there's something we need to learn along the way. There's something (or some things) we need to do as part of the healing process.

Salvation works the same way. God saves us instantly at the moment we give our lives to him. That's when we're born again. Yet we still have to "work out our salvation with fear and trembling," as it says in the book of Philippians. That doesn't mean we save ourselves; we can't do that. It does mean having enough reverence for God and his word that we walk in obedience to him.

For me, being healed, being saved from compulsive overeating has been a process. It's been a struggle. It's been me having to take the long way 'round, having to learn things about myself and about how to live according to God's will. And I'm still not all the way there. I may never be, not until I step out of this life and into the presence of God.

This process of learning obedience means that I'm learning to give up self-will. It often means I have to pray for willingness to be obedient to what God wants me to do, because my natural self is rebellious, selfish, and wants to be in control.

Father, make me willing to be obedient to what you want in my life, including how you want me to eat. In Jesus' name, amen.

by Debbie

June 29

See, I am doing a new thing! Now it springs up; do you not perceive it? I am making a way in the wilderness and streams in the wasteland.
Isaiah 43:19

Sometimes, one of the hardest things to become is willing. And that is the very thing that is necessary before I can change. I have to be willing to let God change me—in whatever way he sees fit. You see, when I was eating compulsively, I was doing it as a way of comforting myself. Sometimes I was angry. Sometimes I was unhappy. Sometimes I was frustrated. Sometimes I was afraid. Sometimes I was just plain weary. I used food to make myself feel better when I felt those things, and most of the time I wasn't even aware what I was feeling.

Why? Because the food effectively masked my emotions. That was the point of eating more than I needed. And yet I didn't fully realize that's what I was doing. In order to change so that I was no longer using food like a five-year-old sucking her thumb and holding a security blanket, I had to become willing to change. But something within me wanted to hold onto that security blanket for all I was worth. I knew it was hurting me, that it was holding me back, but I couldn't let go. I didn't *want* to let go.

So I had to pray for willingness. Just a simple prayer, "God, make me willing to do what you want me to do to overcome my addiction to food, to compulsive eating." Not long afterward, I became willing to try. You can do it too. Pray for willingness. I've never known God to say no to that prayer.

Father, thank you for being so faithful. I don't deserve it, but you love me enough anyway to say yes when I ask for your help. Thank you for putting willingness in my heart when I ask for it. In Jesus' name, amen.

by Debbie

June 30

If you love me, keep my commands.
John 14:15

Part of my recovery from compulsive eating is the willingness to abstain from refined sugar. A few weeks after achieving it, I had a dream in which I broke that abstinence by eating a piece of yellow cake. I didn't taste it in the dream, I just saw it and ate it. I had eaten about half of the piece of cake before I realized that by doing so, I was breaking my food plan, the terms of which is an agreement I've made with God.

Yet in the dream I knew I would get abstinent again right away; there was no doubt in my mind that this was a slip, not a full-fledged relapse. What bothered me at the time is that in the dream, eating the cake was so automatic and that I didn't realize what I had done until I was halfway through with it.

When I woke up, I was so glad it wasn't real! What I learned at the time was just how much abstinence meant to me, even after only a few weeks of doing it. It also confirmed for me that abstinence is precious thing. It needs to be guarded, protected, and valued.

Many of us who eat compulsively have reached a point where becoming abstinent in terms of a substance like sugar or abstinent from eating compulsively has become a matter of life and death, because overeating has so negatively impacted our health. That makes it even more imperative that we protect and value it.

Father, help me to stay willing to be obedient to you, to see it as the most important thing in my life, because that's what shows you that I love you. Help me to choose life every time. In Jesus' name, amen.

by Debbie

Cry of Our Hearts

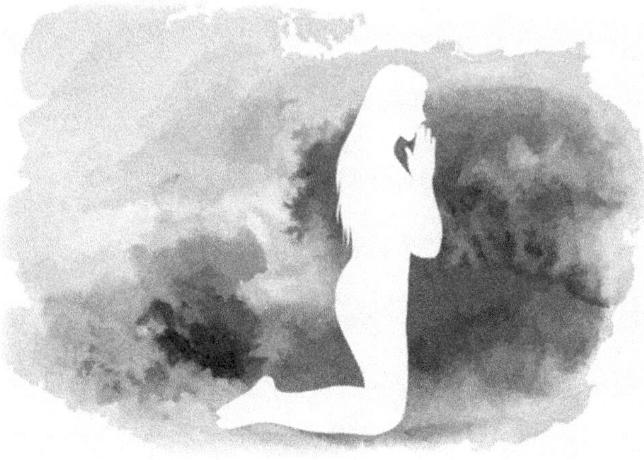

HUMILITY

We ask God to make us better people.

July 1

Humble yourselves, therefore, under the mighty hand of God so that at the proper time he may exalt you, casting all your anxieties on him, because he cares for you.
1 Peter 5:7

God's word tells us to cast all our cares on him. How many times have I cast them all on him and then twenty minutes later taken it back?

How many times have I woken up in the morning and said, "This is the day the Lord has made, and I will follow Him! Lord, today I give my weight-loss efforts to You. I will follow You."

Then by noon I'm trying to figure out what I can do to lose the weight. Maybe if I drink more water. Maybe if I give this or that up. Maybe if I only eat from a small plate. Maybe if I try Weight Watchers.

All those things are good. But are those things what the Lord told *you* to do?

God created each of us to be different. There is no set program that will work for every one of us. That's why it's so important to lay this weight-loss journey at his feet and let him guide you.

Don't fall into the trap of trying to figure it out yourself. That will only lead to frustration. Lay it at his feet and trust him to first show you the way and then to bring you through to the victory!

Can I get a hallelujah?!

Father, help me to stay humble enough to ask for you guidance and direction every day. Help me to be humble enough to accept your instruction. And strong enough to follow it. In Jesus' name, amen.

by Nancy

July 2

Consider it pure joy . . . whenever you face trials of many kinds, because you know that the testing of your faith produces perseverance.
James 1:2–3

Test me, Lord, and try me, examine my heart and my mind.
Psalm 26:2

These past few years have been a trial and a test of my faith in God. In part I have failed, and in part I have passed the test. For those areas where I have failed, I have had to make amends in some way. I also have had to go through a time of learning to overcome compulsive eating. God has led me along the way to bring me closer to what he has in mind for my life. I'm learning to seek him instead of the substitute of food, and I'm learning that instead of living in fear, I can have faith that God will provide everything I need.

I'm learning to ask for confidence instead of living in self-doubt. I'm learning to turn to God to fill the emptiness instead of to food. I'm learning that I can experience negative feelings without having to eat over them, that those feelings pass far more quickly than I often expect.

I'm learning that when I'm tested that it's God who can give me the strength to pass the test. That when I'm tempted, I don't have to give in. That when I feel a compulsion, I don't have to follow it. That God is the strength in me that I could never have on my own.

Father, lead me. Grow me. Help me to continue to surrender to your will. Help me not to fear the humility of failure. Help me to view my life according to biblical principles—as a test and as an exercise in learning to trust. In Jesus' name, amen.

by Debbie

July 3

And the second is like it: you shall love your neighbor as yourself.
Matthew 22:39

When my kids were young, I used to sing to them, "Humble thyself in the sight of the Lord" whenever I felt they were getting big heads. As I got older, I realized it was okay for them to feel good about themselves. To be proud of what they accomplished. I have struggled with that. I find it hard to accept a compliment. I believe the Lord wants us to be humble, but not to the extent that it causes us to not love ourselves.

I'm amazed when I read scriptures that talk about what God sees when he looks at us. Can I pull out a few of those nuggets and apply them to how I feel about myself?

He sees me as his handiwork (Psalm 139:13–16). He sees me as his friend (James 2:23). We radiate light wherever we go (Matthew 5:14). We shine in the night (Philippians 2:15). We are victorious (Romans 8:37). We are chosen by God (John 15:16).

He looks so highly on us. He created each of us to be unique. He has so much good to say about those of us who are his children.

But—can I believe that? Can I start to feel good about myself based on how God sees me? Can I then see that I'm worth working to change for the better? That we can accept what God gives us, just because he loves us so much?

Father, thank you that you have created me to be unique. To be who I am. I don't need to pretend to be something else. I don't need to pretend to be someone else. I just need to love myself and accept all that you say about me. Because what you say is the most important thing. I choose to love myself, to see the beautiful person that you made in the mirror. In Jesus' name, amen.

by Nancy

July 4

You said in your heart, "I will ascend to heaven; above the stars of God. I will set my throne on high; I will sit on the mount of assembly in the far reaches of the north; I will ascend above the heights of the clouds; I will make myself like the Most High."
Isaiah 14:13–14 (ESV)

I know God loves me. I believe I have given my life to him, that I am his. But there's this one thing . . . .

One night I was really struggling with being hungry. I kept going back to the cupboard and the refrigerator. I wasn't eating a lot each time, but it doesn't take many extra calories to make a person gain weight. I'm still trying to lose more weight, so I can't afford any extra trips to the kitchen. I finally cried out to God (which I should have done when the compulsion started), and he showed me that I was unhappy about something and that I was physically tired at the same time. That's a deadly combination, sure to make me reach for my favorite comfort: food.

The next morning, as I was praying to do better that day than I had the night before, God showed me something else. That night I had put myself back on the throne of my own life. I wasn't yielding my will to him. Instead, I was reaching for something familiar for comfort instead of reaching out to him in full submission. I was shocked to realize that made me no different than Lucifer, son of the morning, who still aspires to take God's throne. Thank God the difference is that I don't want to keep doing that. I want to be different, to do God's will. I really do love him and belong to him, but he does want my obedience.

Father, thank you for showing me the truth. Help me to get off the throne and put you back on it where you belong. In Jesus' name, amen.

by Debbie

July 5

When pride comes, then comes disgrace, but with humility comes wisdom.
Proverbs 11:2

The meaning of to follow is: *to go or come after. To move or travel behind.* If God is leading me, I'll be guided in ways that will help my life be better. It won't be perfect, but he'll lead me where I need to be. He'll guide me through the night. He'll shine his light ahead of me. He'll keep me calm.

When I follow, it's not one-sided. He wants me to follow him, but I also *want* to follow him. It's not out of diligence or to have that brief sense of satisfaction. It's a deep-down, in-your-gut understanding that life would not be life without him.

So the real question should be: Do I want brief satisfaction (the kind I get from eating food for comfort), or do I want a lasting relationship with God?

There are a lot of questions I need to ask myself. Have I treated God like he's some special occasion? Have I put what I need into our relationship? Or is it one-sided? Do I only pay attention to him when something bad happens? Do I only notice him when it is convenient for me? Do I only notice him when I want to put on a good show at church? Do I pay attention to him in my quiet moments at home? Do I seek him out when no one is around to watch? Or has it become a "show" of how godly I am?

The thing that comes to my mind is: Humble thyself in the sight of the Lord.

Father, keep my thoughts and motives pure. Help me to follow you with humility and because of a desire to know you more. In Jesus' name, amen.

by Nancy

July 6

I will boast all the more gladly about my weaknesses,
so that Christ's power may rest on me.
2 Corinthians 12:9

"Let the one who boasts boast about this: that they have the understanding to know me, that I am the Lord, who exercises kindness, justice, and righteousness on earth, for in these I delight," declares the Lord.
Jeremiah 9:24

Sometimes when I boast about how well I'm doing with my eating or weight loss, or if I talk about something that worked for me in that area, it's not long after that I get attacked in that very area. It's like the Lord is either working hard to keep me humble, or he's testing me to see if I really meant what I said.

A case in point: I was sharing with friends that I had started doing devotional reading at night expressly to help me with an ongoing difficulty with wanting to eat again at bedtime. It happens when I'm tired, when I've let down my guard, and when my mind is active before I fall asleep. That very night I was tempted again, even *after* doing my spiritual reading.

But then I took an action I have often recommended, which is to **pray through it**. Just a brief prayer: "Lord, help me. I can't do this on my own." And I waited for that false hungry feeling to pass. God is so faithful! The feeling passed quickly. I now understand how God's power is made perfect in my weakness. And I'm oh so grateful to him for doing for me what I cannot do for myself.

Thank you, God. You really are a wonderful Father to me, the weakest of your creatures. In Jesus' name, amen.

by Debbie

July 7

Those who consider themselves religious and yet do not keep a tight rein on their tongues deceive themselves, and their religion is worthless.
James 1:26

Find me in the river
Find me on my knees
I've walked against the water
Now I'm waiting if you please
We've longed to see the roses
But never felt the thorns
And bought our pretty crowns
But never paid the price

A few weeks ago my pastor introduced a new song during worship: "Find Me in the River" (by the band Delirious?). I've played that song a thousand times: *Oh, God, find me in the river on my knees with my soul laid bare.*

It makes me realize that I don't want to put on a show. I don't want people to think how "holy" I am. Oh, God, you're the only one who matters. You're the only one I'm waiting for.

We live in such weird times. How many times have I looked around and become caught up in all the junk happening that I see in the news? In my life? I want to say, "I've got this." No, I do not! GOD has this. Am I willing to let him have it all? Am I willing to be laid bare?

Father, there have been so many times that you have stripped me bare, because you wanted me to rely only on you. Lord, I'm willing to learn from those times. I'm willing to accept this humility so that you can be strong where I am weak. In Jesus' name, amen.

by Nancy

July 8

I can do all things through Him who strengthens me.
Philippians 4:13 NASB

What ways do you think God can help you in your weaknesses—with food or whatever it is you're struggling with right now? One of the ways God profoundly helped me is to remove my terrible temper. When my kids were young, I was irritated easily, and I lost my temper regularly, including yelling, and sometimes I even gave in to rages. I finally realized I had to stop, that I was causing damage to my kids, so I asked God to help, and he took it away. I still got angry sometimes, and I still raised my voice on occasion, but the rages stopped.

Another weakness I asked God to remove was my craving for refined sugar and artificial sweeteners. I've been sugar free for about two years now and free of artificial sweeteners for about a year. Sweet tastes come from fruit and unsweetened juices now. And it's such a blessing! I pray for that to continue one day at a time. I pray I never have to go back to it.

Giving up sugar was a point of obedience to God for me. That's because refined sugar makes me hungrier for everything else. It makes me overeat. Without it, my appetite is regulated, and I can get by with eating less. I want less food when I leave refined sugar out of my diet. Not only that, but I think my rages were connected to my sugar addiction in ways that I can't even fathom.

Thank you, God, for helping me to overcome my fears and step out in faith. Thank you for honoring all my hard work and obedience by giving me the strength to continue doing what you want me to do. Please help me, in my weakness, to keep walking in obedience to your will. In Jesus' name, amen.

by Debbie

July 9

Now we see how God does make us acceptable to him. The Law and the Prophets tell how we become acceptable, and it isn't by obeying the Law of Moses. God treats everyone alike. He accepts people only because they have faith in Jesus Christ. All of us have sinned and fallen short of God's glory. But God treats us much better than we deserve, and because of Christ Jesus, he freely accepts us and sets us free from our sins.
Romans 3:21–24 CEV

Do you identify as fat? As a failure? Or even as a success?

Do you feel like you don't belong anywhere? That your weight, your addiction, holds you back from doing things with your family? That your family and friends don't understand what you're going through? That you just don't fit in?

When I go somewhere, I'm always tempted to look around and see if anyone else is as heavy as I am. Somehow it brings me comfort if there's someone else there who's about my weight. So, again, how are we identifying ourselves? I know that too often I identify more with the fat and the failure.

I was listening to a song the other day, and part of the lyrics ask where my identity is. I've really thought about that.

I need to find my identity in the Lord. When people look at me, they need to see Christ in me. I believe if we just focus on doing that, then we'll start to see ourselves in a better light. I need to take the focus off myself and put it where it belongs.

Father, as I take this time to ask myself the hard questions about my identity, please show me exactly who I am in you. Lord, help me take the focus off myself and put it on you. Let all the other things fall into place. In Jesus' name, amen.

by Nancy

July 10

God is our refuge and strength, an ever-present help in trouble.
Psalm 46:1

Surely God is my salvation; I will trust and not be afraid.
The Lord, the Lord himself, is my strength and my defense;
he has become my salvation.
Isaiah 12:2

The truth is that I don't have the strength on my own to live the Christian life. Nor do I have the strength to eat the way I need to eat to finally reach a healthy body weight. In this way, God means for me to be humble; he wants to ensure that I can't boast about how I can do things on my own.

The truth is that I must ask the Holy Spirit for strength to do God's will. And I have no doubt that it is God's will that I learn to eat in a healthy way, that I learn to depend on God rather than on food as my comfort.

I can ask him to give me the strength and ability to develop a practice and discipline of healthy eating and in the right amounts. I can ask him to help me when I get a sudden urge to eat food that my body doesn't need.

I also need the Spirit to build my faith, and the power of God to do what he has promised, which is to heal me bodily, emotionally, and spiritually.

Father, Lord of All Creation, I humbly ask you to help me today to desire you first above all else. Strengthen me in the places where I am most weak. Take my weakness and give me your strength so I may do your will today. In Jesus' name, amen.

by Debbie

July 11

I've been thinking about my words lately, so I decided to see what God says about them. Sometimes God gives it to me straight, no skirting around. Here's what he wants me to take to heart:

Proverbs 18:21: *The tongue has the power of life and death, and those who love it will eat its fruit.*

Proverbs 29:20: *Do you see a man who speaks in haste? There is more hope for a fool than for him.*

Matthew 12:36–37: *But I tell you that men will have to give account on the day of judgment for every careless word they have spoken. For by your words you will be acquitted, and by your words you will be condemned.*

Matthew 15:11: *What goes into a man's mouth does not make him unclean, but what comes out of his mouth, that is what makes him unclean.*

Matthew 15:18: *But the things that come out of the mouth come from the heart, and these make a man unclean.*

Luke 6:45: *The good man brings good things out of the good stored up in his heart, and the evil man brings evil things out of the evil stored up in his heart. For out of the overflow of his heart his mouth speaks.*

Ephesians 4:29: *Do not let any unwholesome talk come out of your mouths, but only what is helpful for building others up according to their needs, that it may benefit those who listen.*

1 Peter 3:10: *For, whoever would love life and see good days must keep his tongue from evil and his lips from deceitful speech.*

Through his word, God is humbling me. Making me honest. Making sure that my mouth lines up with what I truly want out of this weight-loss journey. If I want victory, then I must speak victoriously!

Father, help me build myself up rather than tear myself down. Amen.

by Nancy

July 12

The Lord works out everything to its proper end.
Proverbs 16:4

The Lord will fulfill his purpose for me; your steadfast love, O Lord, endures forever. Do not forsake the work of your hands.
Psalm 138:8

Remember the former things of old; for I am God, and there is no other; I am God, and there is none like me, declaring the end from the beginning and from ancient times things not yet done, saying, "My counsel shall stand, and I will accomplish all my purpose."
Isaiah 46:10

My life has no purpose apart from God. It's not about me. It's about him. In the past I have always feared seeking my ultimate purpose in God, because I feared losing control of my own life. I feared he would ask me to do something, or many things, that I didn't want to do.

It has only been after many, many years of repeated failure that I have recognized that my way has not been the best way. His way has always been the best way. My job now is to ask him to help me to trust him fully. To ask him to show me his will and then to give me the strength to do it. That is the way I can trust him best. This point of view doesn't exclude the food I eat. For someone like me, for whom food can be a problem, I also must turn that part of my life over to God.

Father, I humble myself before you. I have failed so often, I have no pride left. Help me to live out your purposes for my life, and if that includes following a plan of eating that you want me to follow, then help me to accept that and do it. In Jesus' name, amen.

by Debbie

July 13

He heals the brokenhearted and binds up their wounds.
Psalm 147:3

Weight loss starts in the mind and spirit. If we can't get our minds wrapped up in God and the truth, then we won't see the extra weight come off. We can fake it for a while, but it will come back. The same deep issues will be there.

God longs so much for us to just ask him for what we need. To be our guide, our shepherd. As we turn to the Lord, as we totally trust in the way he leads us, then the true victory will come.

Are you willing to allow God to change you? That can be a scary proposition. People don't want to deal with things they've buried. We'd rather leave them where they are. But what we don't realize is that often those things are festering. They're causing an infection in our minds and with our self-perception. They're wreaking havoc in our family life. In all we do. They can cause a sadness we cover up in front of people. But at home in the dark the feelings come out.

Have you asked God to do surgery on you? Have you asked him to do what needs to be done to get the weight off? Do you know the Lord doesn't need a scalpel? He can heal through his word alone. He is that powerful. How can we ever doubt that we have the key to victory right there in our hearts?

We need to be willing to allow God to dig into what's ailing us. Bring it out. Bring in the healing we need. When our mind is lined up and ready to accept the weight loss and the victory, we'll no longer be negative about the journey. Instead, we'll be free to accept all the good the Lord has planned for us.

Father, I'm willing to let you do surgery on me. Heal me now. Amen.

by Nancy

July 14

This is what the Lord says: "Let not the wise boast of their wisdom or the strong boast of their strength or the rich boast of their riches."
Jeremiah 29:23

One of the things I'm called upon to do as a Christian is to let God work in me, to remove those defects of character that cause me to sin (as in "missing the mark"). One of the things I must always be on guard against in my own life is my tendency to think I know better. Better than others. Sometimes even better than God.

If I rely on my own wisdom, in reality I'm being foolish. Now, I'm a well-educated person, and school always came easy to me. I don't find teaching hard, either. So it's really easy for me to think I know better than other people. And it's even possible to sometimes fool myself into thinking I know better than God. But a little knowledge is often a dangerous thing. And sometimes God's wisdom is exactly the opposite of what we might expect.

That's especially true when it comes to losing weight. How many times have we heard that we just need willpower? But the truth is that willpower doesn't work when it comes to addiction. Relying on a power greater than myself to restore me to sanity is the only thing that has worked for me.

I never thought I was "insane." I thought my life was pretty decent and that I had things in good order. But I now recognize the insanity of allowing my body to be more than a hundred pounds overweight. That's insanity, because it leads to all kinds of health problems. God's way is so much better than mine.

Father, thank you for keeping me humble. Help me to always remember that I can turn to you whenever I need your wisdom. In Jesus' name, amen.

by Debbie

July 15

"Then the lion said, 'You will have to let me undress you.' I was afraid of his claws . . . but I was pretty nearly desperate now. The very first tear he made was so deep that I thought it had gone right into my heart. And when he began pulling the skin off, it hurt worse than anything . . . The only thing that made me able to bear it was just the pleasure of feeling the stuff peel off . . . it must have been a dream."
"No." said Edmund. "You have been—well, un-dragoned."
Eustace in The Voyage of the Dawn Treader *by C. S. Lewis*

Sometimes the Lord needs to peel away our layers. Through this journey I've been shocked at how much needed to be dealt with in my life. The Lord would peel away one thing and then he would show me another area. Then he would peel that away.

Sometimes we have a strong odor, like an onion. And tears fill our eyes as he pulls off the layers. And yet another layer is revealed that has to be dealt with. Then that brings more tears. We're saddened by how much has crept into our lives that we didn't even realize had been buried. And then it festered.

As he peels each layer away, instead of feeling sorrow at what is revealed, I should be glad. I'm glad that he's willing to peel it away. Yes, it may cause me to shed tears. It may cause me to fall on my knees and repent. It could cause some momentary pain. But I can't allow the stink to remain.

It's time to spray the sweet perfume of Jesus on what has become infected and allow the healing to flow through me. As I allow each layer to be peeled, at some point there will be no more to peel away. Victory is coming! I must keep my eye on the prize!

Lord, it's okay with me. I'm ready. I'm at the end of myself. There's nothing left to feel shame about. Peel away the things that need to go. Amen.

by Nancy

July 16

That which has been born of the flesh is flesh,
and that which has been born of the Spirit is spirit.
John 3:6 NASB

In all these things we are more than conquerors through him who loved us.
Romans 8:37

People who have what is often politely termed "a weight problem" know exactly what is meant by "the flesh." Many of us literally live within a lot of flesh every day. What it means in scripture, simply, is our body or our human nature or both.

Scripture tells us we have no choice but to work to overcome the dictates of the flesh. What I've realized about people who have an addiction to food, like me, is that we're intimately connected to the flesh in both ways. We're often ruled by our physical hungers and allergies to food and to the habits with food that we learned in childhood. We're also governed by our human nature, which so often seeks to remove all pain from our lives.

How often have I been dominated by my hungers, whether they were physical or emotional? I was—for most of my adult life. But the Bible also tells me that I can conquer my own flesh—my own hungers—because of what Christ did for me. But I have to reach out and take hold of his strength. It's only in weakness that I can conquer. God has used my weaknesses so that I have no choice but to depend on him. Asking him to change me physically, mentally, emotionally, and spiritually is the only thing that has worked for me. And I have had to be obedient to do what he asked me to do.

Father, thank you for doing for me what I couldn't do in my own power. In Jesus' name, amen.

by Debbie

July 17

Cast all your anxiety on him because he cares for you.
1 Peter 5:7

Come to me, all you who are weary and burdened, and I will give you rest.
Take my yoke upon you and learn from me, for I am gentle
and humble in heart, and you will find rest for your souls.
For my yoke is easy and my burden is light.
Matthew 11:28–30

I was watching a reality TV show called *Brat Camp* where the kids were speaking to an empty chair. At some point, we've all had to do the same, because we haven't been able to speak to the person who hurt us. Maybe we had to go to a cemetery and speak over a grave. Write a letter. Or talk to an empty chair.

One of the girls made a statement that really hit me. Facing the empty chair, she spoke to a man who molested her as a child. She said she was taking back her power. She'd let him have power over her for too long, and she wasn't going to allow it anymore.

As I watched, I was sobbing. I have given other people too much power in my life. I've released the power of past abuses, but I still do it when I worry about my kids. When I wonder what I did wrong as a mother. When I wonder what I could have done differently. Then I have eaten over the stress.

When I give in to those thoughts, they control me. I have to take back that power. I can only do that by turning over my thoughts, my emotions, my worries, my problems to Jesus. To have freedom, I must cast my cares upon him.

Father, help me to forgive myself as well as others. In my humility, help me to find rest in you and to cast my worries on your shoulders. Amen.

by Nancy

July 18

For those God foreknew he also predestined to be conformed to the image of his Son, that he might be the firstborn among many brothers and sisters.
Romans 8:29

One of the ways I can stay on this path, this weight-loss (and weight-maintenance) journey is by allowing God to change me. What I've discovered along the way (along with a lot of others before me) is that I can't pick and choose which things about my character that God is going to change. He chooses.

That helps keep me humble. I can ask God to help me change, but I have no power to actually do the changing myself. The other day, I read:

I need to accept being human and fallible. . . . I don't get to choose which defects God will remove. I find that living with my defects continues to teach me humility. I find that the defects that made me an active threat to society were pretty much removed at once when I stopped my addictive chemical use. . . . God lets me keep the rest of the defects to remind me of my need for daily spiritual contact. They remind me that there is a God, and it isn't me. (Bill P., Todd W., and Sara S. in Drop the Rock.*)*

That means I'll continue on in my human weakness until God takes me home to heaven. I've come to understand that that's a good thing. It's like St. Paul's thorn in the flesh . . . God's grace is sufficient. And it's my weakness that keeps me humble.

Father, thank you for loving me even in my weakness and human frailty. You have a purpose for it. Help me to accept that and to accept myself the way I am. In Jesus' name, amen.

by Debbie

July 19

We bow our hearts
We bend our knees
Oh Spirit come make us humble
We turn our eyes from evil things
Oh Lord we cast out our idols
Give us clean hands
Give us pure hearts
Let us not lift our souls to another
Give us clean hands
Oh God let us be a generation that seeks
Who seeks Your face
Oh God of Jacob
Give us clean hands
"Give Us Clean Hands" *by Charmaine*

Clean hands. I love that song. I was thinking as I was listening to this song, *Have I bowed my heart and knees? Have I lifted my soul to something other than God? Maybe food? Greediness?*

There are so many sins that come with being overweight. Oh, sure, I don't like to think like that, but it's the truth.

I can bow my heart and bend my knee for other things. What about in the area of my eating? Am I pure in that area? Can I choose to bow my head and bend my knee when it comes to the choices I make with food?

Oh, God, let me seek your face. Oh, God, give me clean hands. Make me humble, Lord. Let me seek to do your will when it comes to everything in my life, including the food I put in my body. In Jesus' name, amen.

by Nancy

July 20

For he chose us in him before the creation of the world
to be holy and blameless in his sight.
Ephesians 1:4

The Lord your God is with you, the Mighty Warrior who saves.
He will take great delight in you; in his love he will no longer
rebuke you, but will rejoice over you with singing.
Zephaniah 3:17

For a long time, shame was a defining influence in my life. It came from sinful actions I took as a young woman that had dire consequences. As a result, I was ashamed of myself, and I was shamed before others. One of the gifts of this weight-loss journey has been to see myself as I really am. To recognize that I'm no different from anyone else. We all fall short. We all have things we've done that we could or should be ashamed of.

No longer do I need to hide my past, hide in shame. In human terms, that past occurred long ago, and I have lived a different kind of life for a long time. One that I can be proud of in terms of making different choices, better choices. If I hadn't learned from the past, that would be one thing, but I did learn, and I changed. I'm not perfect, but I'm better. Wiser.

One thing I learned is that I no longer need to live in shame. That's because Jesus bore my shame on the cross, and he looks at me now and sees me as blameless. He paid the price, and he no longer rebukes me, because he has already forgiven me.

Father, thank you and praise you for the amazing gift of your Son, who took my shame and paid the price for it so that you could count me as righteous. In Jesus' name, amen.

by Debbie

July 21

Your beauty should not come from outward adornment, such as elaborate hairstyles and the wearing of gold jewelry or fine clothes. Rather, it should be that of your inner self, the unfading beauty of a gentle and quiet spirit, which is of great worth in God's sight.
1 Peter 3:3–4

The Lord does not look at the things people look at. People look at the outward appearance, but the Lord looks at the heart.
1 Samuel 16:7

Perhaps if we lived in another culture, women "of size" would be revered, because it means we're "wealthy." Unfortunately, we live in a culture that worships thin.

I once knew someone who probably was thin her whole life. In all likelihood, she never struggled with it. I always got the unspoken message from her that she thought she was better than I was. Sadly, we live in a world in which that happens far too often. But what if we don't buy into that anymore? Not that we should accept being an *unhealthy* weight, but as we're learning what it takes to lose weight and keep it off permanently, why do we have to feel horrible about the way we look?

Are those people really better than we are? God says no, they're not. All of us fall short. All of us sin. None of us are worthy on our own. It's only in Christ, through his sacrifice on the cross, through the shedding of his blood, that we become worthy, that we become children of God. May we learn to walk in that truth.

Father, help me to see my true worth through your eyes, not the eyes of the culture around me. In Jesus' name, amen.

by Nancy

July 22

The fear of the Lord is a fountain of life,
turning a person from the snares of death.
Proverbs 14:27

Teach us to number our days,
that we may gain a heart of wisdom.
Psalm 90:12

I've been unwise for a good portion of my life. I look back at my younger years, when I made several unwise decisions that led to lasting consequences. Since then, one of my ongoing prayers has been to ask God to give me wisdom and discernment.

One of the areas where I've been unwise is with eating and food. I was like a kid in a candy store. Once I became an adult, I loved that I could choose what, when, where, and how much I ate. I so loved being in control that I spun completely out of control! Because of that, I now understand what God meant when he said, "The wages of sin is death." I made decisions, and I'm now paying the wages for them. I might not be dying physically (today), but there have been consequences for eating unwisely for so many years that have impacted my quality of life.

Yet even while living in those consequences, I can be grateful. Why? Because God is gracious and merciful. Though sin produces death, God can "restore the years the locusts have eaten." Once I stepped back into obedience, he blessed me mightily. He will do that for anyone who turns around (repents) and walks in a new direction.

Father, thank you for restoration and renewal and for sometimes reversing the deadly consequences of sin, even in this life. In Jesus' name, amen.

by Debbie

July 23

You're cheating on God. If all you want is your own way, flirting with the world every chance you get, you end up enemies of God and his way. And do you suppose God doesn't care? The proverb has it that "he's a fiercely jealous lover." And what he gives in love is far better than anything else you'll find. It's common knowledge that "God goes against the willful proud; God gives grace to the willing humble." So let God work his will in you. Yell a loud no to the devil and watch him scamper. Say a quiet yes to God, and he'll be there in no time. Quit dabbling in sin. Purify your inner life. Quit playing the field. Hit bottom and cry your eyes out. The fun and games are over. Get serious, really serious. Get down on your knees before the Master; it's the only way you'll get on your feet.
James 4:4–10 The Message

There have been times when I'm in a funk with my weight loss, when I'm at the point of struggling with wanting to give up. At those times, God gives me nudges to keep going.

The reading above from *The Message* really spoke to me. Sometimes it's easier to think, "God doesn't care." But his word says otherwise. It calls him a jealous lover. It tells us to be healthy.

So if I'm choosing food over him, then he's jealous of that. And what he wants to give me is far better even than what I want for myself. I so often think the food is good *now*. But in the long run, what God has is much better. If I can just take my eyes off the present and look to the long term, just maybe I'll make it.

Father, thank you for caring enough about me to push me when I want to give up. Thank you for being jealous of my time and attention—it shows me you love me. Maybe you have given me these struggles with weight to keep me humble, and to keep my eyes on you. Help me to be "willfully humble" before you. In Jesus' name, amen.

by Nancy

July 24

Then you will call, and the Lord will answer;
you will cry for help, and he will say: Here am I.
Isaiah 58:9

If I had cherished sin in my heart, the Lord would not have listened.
Psalm 66:18

I've tried this weight-loss journey many times, and I've been a part of a twelve-step program twice, with about a dozen years between each attempt. I lost about seventy pounds the first time around. In the terminology of twelve-step programs, that means I had a long "relapse" during which I gained back most of the weight I had lost. What caused the relapse? Me not putting a high priority on spiritual growth. Oh, I went to church. I believed in God and in his Son Jesus. But I did not have a daily devotional time, and I didn't ask God to help me with my weight loss.

But it was more than that. It isn't just about being fat. It's about not turning every part of my life over to the care of God. If I'm holding onto my food, which I was—as tightly as I could grasp it—then I haven't surrendered everything, have I? Like the Psalm says, I was cherishing my sin—my love affair with food. And when I do that, it's clear that the Lord doesn't listen. Yet now when I cry out for help, the Lord listens *and* answers.

What's the difference? When I make obedience to him my priority, when I do things his way instead of mine—including my food choices—then God listens, he answers, and I have success.

Father, keep me humble. Help me to see that your way is the better way—that my way leads to defeat and failure. Help me to understand that you know what's best for me and help me to accept what you want. In Jesus' name, amen.

by Debbie

July 25

But the things that come out of a person's mouth
come from the heart, and these defile them.
Matthew 15:18

Wow—the things I've said to myself are coming from my heart. I needed to let that soak in. Are the feelings I have for myself only negative? I see the answer as a kind of heart surgery. The only way I know for that to happen is to spend more time with God. He is the only one who can fix what is in my heart that has allowed me to grow so cold toward myself. I need to allow him to do the work that needs to be done.

Mending the heart is never easy. But it will be worth it. I think about how good that sounds to not have so much hate for myself. To see myself as God does. That would be so amazing. So freeing. So . . . light. Like a weight taken off. Could it happen? If I allow God to fix my heart, could the weight problem be fixed too? I think about my grandkids. I hate it when they say something negative about themselves. It breaks my heart. I want them to know just how wonderful they are. How smart they are. How beautiful and handsome they are.

Isn't that what God wants for me? Does it break his heart to hear me say bad things about myself? He loves me so much more than I could possibly understand. So I'll reach out to him. Grab onto him. He's used to tight holds. I'll hang on tight and allow him to do what needs to be done. I'll ask him to let me see myself as he does.

Father, there's a wrong kind of humility—humiliation—and right kind of humility—being humble. Let me not humiliate myself but instead be humble enough to accept your love. In Jesus' name, amen.

by Nancy

July 26

Why spend money on what is not bread, and your labor on what does not satisfy? Listen, listen to me, and eat what is good, and you will delight in the richest of fare.
Isaiah 55:2

It seems funny to use this scripture here, because aren't we trying to avoid rich fare? As we work to lose weight, that's entirely true. But I don't think this verse is actually referring to food. Or if it is, it has a dual meaning. What I see here is the idea that it's only God who satisfies. Jesus said, "Do not work for food that spoils, but for food that endures to eternal life . . . I am the bread of life. Whoever comes to me will never go hungry."

This has been one of the hardest lessons for me to learn, probably because I've turned to food for so long instead. What I have learned along the way is that when I do turn to God he does satisfy my longing. And his word backs that up:

For he satisfies the longing soul,
and the hungry soul he fills with good things.
Psalm 107:9

Father, when I feel empty, I know my soul is actually longing for you. Most of the time I don't understand that. I think I want something else and I so often reach for it. Please remind me. Help me to remember that it's you who satisfies. I truly want to turn to you when I'm feeling false hunger. Because I'm not really hungry for food then, am I? Lord, I fall short so often, yet you have said in your word that you will satisfy my longing soul. Help me to turn to you, in humility, instead of to the false idol of food—or anything else—to receive everything you have to give. In Jesus' name, amen.

by Debbie

July 27

I know your deeds, that you are neither cold nor hot.
I wish you were either one or the other! So, because you are lukewarm
—neither hot nor cold—I am about to spit you out of my mouth.
Revelation 3:15–16

One thing you learn when you have a chronic illness is that you can't talk about it. You can't tell people how you're feeling. You can rarely be real. So often you just have to fake it. That's because so many Christians will say, "You have to have faith. You're not believing enough. Have you even asked for healing?" And so on, blah blah blah.

I'd like to give some advice to the people with such horrible advice: "Don't waste your breath. My soul has been laid bare. It's cracked and dry. And God still loves me. He hears my thoughts. He hears my heart. My words, your words, are nothing." That's because God is sovereign. He can use my suffering. It may be for my good. Or for someone else's. He never told us that once we became Christians everything would be hunky-dory. In fact, he told us that we would suffer right along with the rest of the world.

The biggest thing to learn from this fake Christianity is to realize that we're not pulling anything over God's eyes. He hears. He sees. God sees your heart. He hears your thoughts, the cold or the hot. It's important to serve him with your heart, not just your mouth.

Father, help me always remember that you are God, you are King, and I am not. Keep me humble enough to remember that you know what you're doing and how often I don't know anything at all. Then remind me that I need to follow you, to choose what you want instead of what I want. And please make your people more understanding about chronic illness. In Jesus' name amen.

by Nancy

July 28

Oh, the depth of the riches of the wisdom and knowledge of God!
How unsearchable his judgments, and his paths beyond tracing out!
Who has known the mind of the Lord? Or who has been his counselor?
Who has ever given to God, that God should repay them?
Romans 11:33–35

In my attempts to lose weight, it's been important to keep perspective. I often think of a scene from the movie *Rudy* in which he is seeking advice from a priest about his seemingly impossible desire to play football at Notre Dame University. Rudy asks, "Can you help me?" The priest answers, "Son, in thirty-five years of religious studies, I've come up with only two hard, incontrovertible facts: There is a God. And . . . I'm not him."

For years I tried to lose weight without addressing its true cause: the compulsion to overeat. As a Christian, I shake my head that it wasn't my first, second, or even my third thought that I should seek God's help. A huge part of my failing to turn to God with it is because I enjoyed overeating. It was fun. Even now I have to be careful not to dwell on memories of the pleasures of certain foods. I've heard that sometimes with drug addiction, the pleasure that was there at first is eventually gone. That hasn't been true with food, and I don't know that will ever happen.

What I've learned is that to overcome this weakness that has become such an ingrained part of me, I have to reach out to God in humility, recognizing that I'm the creature and he is the Creator. That means he knows best, and I'd better try it his way instead of mine. He is God, and I'm not him.

Father, help me to recognize your truth because it is *the truth. Give me the willingness to let go of my way and to walk in your way instead. Amen.*

by Debbie

July 29

I will give them a heart to know Me, for I am the LORD;
and they will be My people, and I will be their God,
for they will return to Me with their whole heart.
Jeremiah 24:7 NKJV

Self-worth. This is a huge subject when it comes to weight loss and so many other things in my life. Does my self-worth lie in the fat? This can even pertain to my job. Does my self-worth lie in what level I attain at work? Where do I put my self-worth?

I wonder, where does *God* want me to put my self-worth?

I often focus so much on the day-to-day stuff. I focus on my weight, because I can't find anything to wear. What will people think of this outfit? My mind whirls. The gears keep turning. Think, think, think. Sometimes my mind takes me to places that I should never go. God would much rather my focus be on his word. What does *he* think? Where does *he* want me to go? What steps does *he* want me to take today?

How I start my day can make such a difference. Do I start it with a prayer and a word from the Lord? Or do I start it with rush rush rush? Even if it means getting up just a bit earlier, it's well worth the time to just sit and have a cup of coffee with God. He has a whole new world he wants to open up to me.

Father, I pray that I would open my heart and really take the time to get to know you. Lord, help me to find the perfect time to just sit and visit with you. A time of refreshing. A time of learning. And a time of just being with you. Please make each person reading this now grow in her knowledge of you. Give each of them a heart overflowing with you and your love. In Jesus' name, amen.

by Nancy

July 30

Shout for joy to the Lord, all the earth. Worship the Lord with gladness; come before him with joyful songs. Know that the Lord is God. It is he who made us, and we are his; we are his people, the sheep of his pasture. Enter his gates with thanksgiving and his courts with praise; give thanks to him and praise his name. For the Lord is good and his love endures forever; his faithfulness continues through all generations.
Psalm 100

There is so much to be grateful for in recovery from any addiction, including to compulsive eating. In fact, doing the things I need to do to walk in recovery are part of what makes me so full of gratitude, especially for how God has changed me and is continuing his work in me and in my life. I've learned how to take responsibility for my own actions; to make amends when I've done something wrong; to turn to God instead of to the comfort of food; to be more honest with myself, God, and others; and the true meaning of daily surrender. I don't do it perfectly, but I'm learning, and I'm making progress.

Some of the things I'm grateful for are how patient the Lord is with me. How kind and loving he is. How he takes care of my needs, sometimes even before I know to ask. How he delights sometimes in surprising me with things that delight my heart (like a beautiful sunset or catching a glimpse of a baby bunny feeding among the flowers in a garden, or—best of all—finding out that I'm finally going to become a grandmother).

It's only in humility that I can be grateful, because it's only by acknowledging that I can't gain these things on my own that I have learned to be thankful to the one who can give them: God.

Father, I praise and thank you for your many, many blessings. Amen.

by Debbie

July 31

Refrain from anger and turn from wrath; do not fret—it leads only to evil. For those who are evil will be destroyed, but those who hope in the Lord will inherit the land.
Psalm 37:8–9

I had one of those frustrating days. So much happened that made me upset. The first thing just annoyed me. After the second thing, I felt like a huge bomb went off inside me. Then things that happened a week ago came back up in my thoughts that just added to the day's frustration. As the day went on, I noticed I wasn't feeling well. It just kept getting worse. I developed a headache and my neck hurt.

How many times do I stop to think where anger, frustration, or hurt take me? Not only what it does to my emotions, but to my physical body too. I felt like I was deteriorating throughout the day. Now, if I had taken the time to stop and calm down, if I had said a prayer or two, the situation may have been extinguished, it may not have built up to anything more than a small annoyance that went away quickly.

The Lord says if we'll refrain from anger, we'll inherit the land. God knows what unresolved anger can do to me, how it can affect my health. He says many times in his word to refrain from anger. I need to heed his word. Then—more than maybe—I would feel better physically and emotionally.

Father, help me understand what negative emotions do to me and my health. How they can affect my life, my job, and my family. They can make me downright miserable. Help me to learn to go to you first, lay it at your feet, and move forward in my day with the peace that comes from knowing you have it covered, that you'll take care of every situation. In Jesus' name, amen.

by Nancy

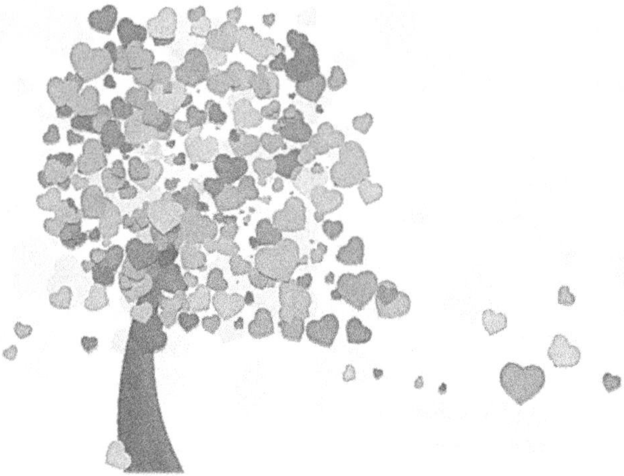

LOVE

We learn how we can
best love God and others.

Cry of Our Hearts

August 1

O God, you are my God, earnestly I seek you; my soul thirsts for you, my body longs for you, in a dry and weary land where there is no water. My soul will be satisfied as with the richest of foods; with singing lips my mouth will praise you.
Psalm 63:1,5

I sat down with my guitar to do a little worship, choosing a song written by a friend. As I was singing, I asked myself if I was really living what I was singing. Part of it says:

Lord I love you, Lord I love you, I worship at your feet and I adore you
Lord my heart pants after thee, no matter who may see
The world means naught to me, I love you with abandon

I was thinking: Does my heart pant after him enough to abandon all the extra food? Would I abandon this bad habit to pant after my Father in heaven? Do I adore him enough to give it all up for him? These questions could go on for many things in our lives. Food? Drugs? Drinking? Overspending?

Another part of the song says:

Oh, the service to her King, though it costs her everything
Is to God a lovely thing, love with abandon

It cost her everything. What a simple thing to give to him: extra helpings, sugar, and so on. Yet it's so hard! But God says he'll give us strength.

I pray that this will be a week that I pant after God and give him all that he deserves, which is my whole life, including my food. In Jesus' name, amen.

by Nancy

August 2

Do not seek revenge or bear a grudge against anyone among your people, but love your neighbor as yourself. I am the LORD.
Leviticus 19:18

No one looked on you with pity or had compassion enough to do any of these things for you. Rather, you were thrown out into the open field, for on the day you were born you were despised.
Ezekiel 16:5

Love your neighbor as yourself. So then do I have any love to give? Do I love myself? Loving myself can sometimes be hard.

That's because abuse left a big sting in my life. I felt as if everyone abandoned me. As if I wasn't worthy of being taken care of. As if I'd been cast out into a field and everybody loathed me. If you have been through divorce, the rejection goes to the core. Should I reject myself, then? If my spouse thought I wasn't worthy of his love or care, why should I? Do you allow others to determine your worth? I know I have. But I need to see that the only one who determines my worth is the Lord. And he thinks I'm worthy of all the good that can come into my life.

Do you see how our feelings about ourselves can determine our weight-loss success? If I feel worthless, rejected, hurt, angry, and bitter with myself, then what is going to make me want to lose the extra weight? If I don't love myself then I'm not going to care enough to do the very best myself.

I can't allow others to determine the person that I am! I must remember that God created me! And he thinks I'm awesome!

Father, thank you for loving me first, even when I wasn't loveable. Please give me the grace to love myself too. In Jesus' name, amen.

by Nancy

August 3

Again, though I say to the wicked, 'You shall surely die,' yet if he turns from his sin and does what is just and right, if the wicked restores the pledge, gives back what he has taken by robbery, and walks in the statutes of life, not doing injustice, he shall surely live; he shall not die. None of the sins that he has committed shall be remembered against him. He has done what is just and right; he shall surely live.
Ezekiel 33:14–16 ESV

How do I show people I love them? One way is to recognize how I might have harmed them. Living in close proximity to someone for any length of time means there's more than a good chance that I've done something or other I need to apologize for, something that I need to make right.

Yet I can't live in guilt, because if I do, it may cause me to overeat. I must deal with my feelings. If I let them fester, I *know* I'll run to food, because that's been my default go-to for a long time. But in learning to take care of business, to make amends when I need to, I also have freedom to move forward. I no longer have to go to my old default position. I can choose a new default.

So, when I've wronged someone, I need to own up to it and make it right. If I've stolen, I need to pay restitution. If I've hurt someone's feelings, I need to admit that to the person's face and apologize, vowing to be more careful with my words in the future. In that way not only do I show love for the person I've harmed, but I also show love to myself, because I've chosen to sweep my side of the street. I've chosen to live in freedom.

Father, when you bring my sins against others to mind, help me to love them best by making things right with them. Then I can be right with you too. In Jesus' name, amen.

by Debbie

August 4

"Though the mountains be shaken and the hills be removed, yet my unfailing love for you will not be shaken nor my covenant of peace be removed," says the Lord, who has compassion on you.
Isaiah 54:10

How do you label yourself? When I think about my past I come up with failure:

I failed at being a daughter. I was into all the wrong things. I was hurtful toward my parents. And on and on.

I failed as a teenager. If you could do it wrong, I was right there doing it.

I failed as a wife. I did so many things wrong in my first marriage. And still do in my second marriage.

I failed at marriage. I have a divorce under my belt.

I failed at mothering. My kids have chosen a rough road. It must have been me, right?

I failed at weight loss. I had a hard time finding a pattern that worked for me.

I'm definitely the hardest on myself.

Is there a way past that? If we look at all that God says about us, we'll once and for all see the truth. There are many places where God talks about how we are the apple of his eye. No matter what you or I have done, we are special in his sight. Aren't you glad that God doesn't label us as harshly as we label ourselves?

Father, help me not to live in my failures. Instead, help me to understand and live in the way that you see me. Then help me to walk in your love. In Jesus' name, amen.

by Nancy

August 5

Mary sat at the Lord's feet listening to what he said.
"Mary has chosen what is better, and it will not be taken away from her."
Luke 10:39,42

I often run to and fro looking for anything that will satisfy what is missing in my life. I also run to food to find satisfaction.

Yet, if I have complete fellowship with the Lord, then I'll be completely satisfied. There's so much waiting for me in the Throne Room if I'll just get to that room more often. I need to sit at his feet and listen to all he has for me. I need to get there and just love on the Father. Oh, how sweet and wonderful it is to just sit at the feet of my Lord and worship him.

When I surrender to him, I'm not looking for anything else to satisfy me. I've found complete satisfaction right there in my prayer closet.

I shouldn't just run to God in a hurry and say, "Oh, Lord, help me" and then run about my daily business. That won't bring the satisfaction that only he can give. I know it doesn't work, because I tried it for years. Only when I truly spent time with the Father did I know what true satisfaction was. I no longer craved a worldly kind of satisfaction.

Money, cars, jobs, food, games, fun, will not bring satisfaction. You'll still feel that something is missing in your life. That something is actually *Someone.*

Lord, remind me to take the time to just go and be with Daddy God today. Let me never forget how amazed I am at how different I come away every time I sit in your presence and just experience the joy of being with you. In Jesus' name, amen.

by Nancy

August 6

Be devoted to one another in love. Honor one another above yourselves.
Romans 12:10

One of the things I didn't realize about giving in to daily compulsive overeating was that it affected the people around me too. I mean, how could my choices about what and how much to eat make any difference to anyone but myself? But they did.

Being heavy meant I couldn't do as many physical things with my kids. It meant that I spent time fixated on food that I could have spent with my family. It meant that sometimes I went into rages—probably induced by a sugar high (or the resulting drop in blood sugar after a sugar binge). It meant I wasn't as attractive as I could have been for my husband. It probably meant a bunch of other things that I still don't even realize.

Even now, I'm paying some consequences for being heavy that may be affecting my family. My weight may have contributed to my back, knee, and hip problems. It means that I can't do as much physically as I might have had I maintained a healthy body weight my entire life. Reflecting on those dismal facts reminds me that this is a serious disease. It's no joke. And it isn't just about me. As I think about that, I have to fight shame and remember that God has forgiven me.

Part of loving the people around me consists of taking care of my body. Part of honoring others above myself means that I need to put aside self-will and eat in a responsible and disciplined way that will keep me healthier. Why? So that I can continue to love the people who need me for as long as possible.

Father, help me to love the people I love by loving myself enough to take care of my health. Help me to eat responsibly. In Jesus' name, amen.

by Debbie

August 7

I will walk among you and be your God, and you will be my people.
Leviticus 26:12

What kind of relationship do you have with God? On some days I feel that I just have a "take" relationship with him. It seems to always be me praying, "God will you do this for me? God, please bless me with this!"

And then I realize that God wants to be my friend too. So then I look at my close friendships. What am I like with them? I talk about my day with them. We discuss hairstyles. We get silly and laugh. And sometimes we cry together.

I've heard it preached that you shouldn't go to God with trivial stuff like choosing your hairstyle for the day. But you know what? I think he wants us to. He wants to be a part of every decision. Every moment of our day. He wants that silly relationship with us. He wants to laugh with us. When we're excited or sad about something, he wants to be the first person we talk to. I sometimes think I have to always try to be perfect with God, and maybe that's what hinders my relationship with him. Maybe he wants me to come as I am and just enjoy a friendship with him.

Some people may see God as harsh, someone or something to be scared of. But he loves you so much. He sees the good and the bad, and yet he still cares. He sees you as the apple of his eye.

So today, instead of calling an earthly friend with my sadness or excitement—or even my hairdo quandary—I'll call God first! I truly believe he would love to hear from me.

Father, I know I can run to you with my big problems, but help me remember that you want to hear about the little things too. In Jesus' name, amen

by Nancy

August 8

Altogether, Enoch lived a total of 365 years. Enoch walked faithfully with God; then he was no more, because God took him away.
Gen 5:23–24

Some days I feel that life is all about dieting. That's all I think on. That's all I breathe. What can I eat today? What should I avoid today? What should I change today so that I can get the weight off? If only I were thinner, these pants would fit better. How can I do my hair so my face looks thinner? The list goes on. Before I know it my whole day has been consumed with dieting—without one thought about what God thinks of any of it.

I truly think that if I would focus my day on the Lord, I would be so consumed by goodness and mercy that at the end of the day I would realize I hadn't thought about dieting at all.

I know I need to think about things going on in my daily life. But just maybe when I'm not dealing with everyday stuff, I can think on him. Maybe when thinking about what to feed my family, I can ask him what he thinks. Sometimes I toss so many ideas around and then suddenly realize I've spent thirty minutes just deciding what to have for supper. That's twenty-nine wasted minutes that could be spent with the Lord.

It's all about him! That's how I need to walk through my days. It's all about him. Not me. Not the diet. Not everything that tries to steal my time away. I'd like to be like Enoch. He walked with God. Maybe when Enoch walked, all people saw was the Lord. Am I willing to be that dedicated to him?

Father, help me be more like Enoch. I want to know what it means to walk with you every day. In Jesus' name, amen.

by Nancy

August 9

Do not seek revenge or bear a grudge against anyone among your people, but love your neighbor as yourself. I am the Lord.
Leviticus 19:18

But he wanted to justify himself, so he asked Jesus, "And who is my neighbor?"
Luke 10:29

My neighbors are the people whose lives I touch. That includes family, friends, my church, and, yes, actual neighbors. One thing I've learned in this weight-loss journey is that part of loving my neighbor means that if I've done something wrong to someone, I need to first admit it and then make it right.

I find that extremely difficult and humbling. Sometimes it's downright scary to think about going to someone—my daughter, say—to ask for forgiveness. Some of the people I have asked have given their forgiveness freely. Others might not—and those are the ones who make me want to procrastinate.

Yet I need to do it anyway. Why? Because unconfessed wrongs, shortcomings, errors—sin—inevitably makes me uncomfortable. And being uncomfortable is what makes me want to eat more. If I don't clear the air, wash my hands, clean my side of the street, I'll be uncomfortable. I like being comfortable. I hate being uncomfortable. I can either do what I need to do to get comfortable again (confess what I did and make amends), or I'll invariably reach for my favorite comfort foods. One of those choices leads to real victory; the other leads to ultimate defeat.

Father, show me when I need to confess my sins and when I need to make amends to the people around me. Then give me the strength. Amen.

by Debbie

August 10

As a bridegroom rejoices over his bride, so will your God rejoice over you.
Isaiah 62:5

Think about your wedding. If you're not married yet, then think about what your dream wedding would be like. Think about the excitement. The anticipation. The joy. It's something you plan for. It's something you work hard for. You do all that you can to make sure it's the perfect day. A day you'll remember forever. It's a special day. A day to cherish. A day to never forget.

You want all the details just right. You study up on different types of weddings. You choose the colors, the flowers. You put special effort into deciding every detail of each part of your special day.

And it's fun. It's not a chore doing all that, because it leads to the most awesome day of your life. You look at the person you're going to marry with such love and admiration. And you want to make sure the day is just as special for him. You see your joy and happiness wrapped up in him for the next hundred years of your life.

The day can't come soon enough. You're on the edge of your seat waiting to celebrate a love for each other that runs deep.

Now imagine that we can have that experience every day of our lives. We can, because we are the bride of Christ. We can pour out the same love and devotion. And Jesus is worth celebrating. He's worth the joy and anticipation of the day we'll meet him face to face. The day that he will come for us, his bride, and we'll get to be with him forever.

Lord, help me to be ready when you come for me. I can't wait! I long for you in the same way a bride longs for her future husband. I love you. Amen.

by Nancy

August 11

"Love your neighbor as yourself."
Mark 12:31

We love because he first loved us.
1 John 4:19

***

I was thinking about the scripture that talks about loving others as we love ourselves. Then I thought about what I once heard a pastor say: that people that are overweight must *reeaallyy* love themselves.

I disagree. Being overweight comes from *not* loving myself enough. Not feeling worthy of taking care of myself. Not feeling that I measure up to the people in my life. I'll often take care of *them.* But I won't take care of myself.

Is there is something within me that I hate so much that I'm willing to commit slow suicide to get rid of it? A self-loathing? I suspect that's true.

If I paid attention to how special I am to God, if I could let it sink in just how precious I am to him, maybe, just maybe, I could love myself enough to get myself healthy.

Genetics plays a part. So does what's going on in my life. But there's also something that God wants to bring to the open to help set me free from what is literally weighing me down.

That tells me it's a hard fight—but I need to remember that God is *glad* to help me. If I'm willing to let him.

Father, let your love overshadow and surround me to the point where I have no choice but to love myself too. And in loving myself and loving you, help me to take the right actions, those that will help me to become healthy in body and spirit so that I can live the way you want me to live. In Jesus' name, amen.

by Nancy

August 12

Your love is more delightful than wine.
Song of Solomon 1:2

Let us rejoice and be glad and give him glory! For the wedding of the Lamb has come, and his bride has made herself ready.
Revelation 19:7

In the Song of Solomon, a picture of the relationship between Christ and his bride, the Church, the bride, says, "Your love is better than wine."

Throughout the Bible, wine is a symbol of earthly pleasure. This imagery makes me think of a lunch out I once had with a couple of friends. One ordered a chocolate cake covered in ice cream and warm melted chocolate. She took a bite and said, "I've died and gone to heaven."

I'm like that. Rather than in wine, my earthly pleasure was always wrapped up in the food I ate. Then, after a while, it was no longer about hunger, but about filling up something that was missing.

God's love is what my heart is really longing for, and I have been using food to fill up that emptiness. What a poor substitute! If I opt for food instead of God's presence, instead of choosing to wrap myself up in his love, it will never satisfy. I will never be satisfied. Not to mention that partaking in food my body doesn't need has dire consequences on my health and well-being.

Father, help me to turn to you, to seek your face and your love. When I think I'm hungry and I'm really not, remind me that you are the one who satisfies. You are the only one who can satisfy my soul. Help me to turn to you instead of to food. In Jesus' name, amen.

by Debbie

August 13

Then they cried out to the Lord in their trouble; He saved them from their distresses. He brought them out of darkness and the shadow of death and broke their bands apart. They shall give thanks to the Lord for His mercy, and for His wonders to the sons of mankind! For He has shattered gates of bronze and cut off bars of iron.
Psalm 107:13–16

This scripture speaks of being brought out of the darkness of prison. Of being set free. I was raped as a teenager. I gave that rapist a good twenty years of my life, and he didn't even know it. I was the one who suffered. I was the one who was in prison for what he did. And there came a time to take back my life.

All of us have one thing or another, maybe many things, that are "weighing" us down. It may have crushed you when it happened. But the time has come to break free. To not give that thing another moment of your time. To not allow the past to rule your life. To take back what is yours. To take back health and happiness. One way to do that is to give your heart fully to God. If you haven't done that, consider doing it now. God loves you so much. He even loves you through your addictions, whether it be gluttony, drugs, alcohol, porn, gambling, or overspending.

God wants to help you. He wants you to reach out to him, find comfort in him. It's simple to say, "God, I'm sorry for what I've done. I need you in my life. Come into my life and help me." He wants to do that for you. He is an awesome Father, and he is faithful.

Father, sometimes I'm controlled by my sins. Sometimes by my trauma. But you have an answer for both. You can forgive my sins. You can heal my trauma. Come into my life with cleansing and healing power. In Jesus' name, amen.

by Nancy

August 14

He has sent me to . . . bestow on them a crown of beauty
instead of ashes, the oil of joy instead of mourning,
and a garment of praise instead of a spirit of despair.
Isaiah 61:1,3

I recently watched an HGTV show called *Home Town*. The husband-and-wife hosts were working on a home for a couple who wanted to use it to house women who needed a fresh start. They may have been homeless or just released from prison.

As they walked through to examine the interior to see what needed to be upgraded and repaired, one item they commented on were the floors. It was easy to see that they were well worn. They were chipped and marred. But as the wife bent down to examine them closely, she remarked about how beautiful they were. They then walked from room to room, and things I thought were not so cute she just oohed and aahed over. She saw the beauty. She then talked about how so many of us are well worn. We may have some cracks. And she wished everyone would show their scars more, because those very flaws are a testament to what someone has been through and won victory over. Those scars make people even more beautiful. The *scars* are beautiful.

A few days ago, some of my family members were together, and several cousins stood up for a group photo. When I saw it later, it hit me hard. I absolutely hated how I looked in it. Yet I wonder if I took the time to look at my "scars" and remember the reason why they're there, then maybe I could see the beauty, fat and all. Then, maybe, everyone else could see it too.

Father, help me to love myself, scars and all. Help me to see the value in the lessons I learned from you through those scars. In Jesus' name, amen.

by Nancy

August 15

You are not your own; you were bought at a price.
Therefore, honor God with your bodies.
1 Corinthians 6:20

As a Christian, I have been aware for a long time that my body is the temple of the Holy Spirit and that I should treat it as such. In some ways I obeyed that idea, but in many others I did not.

The fact is, we do tend to love ourselves. We make sure our needs are met and a lot of our wants too, when we can. So I did love myself—sometimes selfishly. But there were other things that I did, or neglected to do, that showed that I didn't always love myself in a way that truly promotes my overall well-being.

I failed in the type and amounts of food I chose to put in my body, which allowed me to balloon up to my highest weight at 287 pounds. But there were other ways too. I sometimes didn't take good care of my teeth—I brushed them, but we all know that's not enough. I avoided going to the dentist for many years out of fear.

Today, I have put a greater priority on taking better care of my body. I eat far less than I used to, and I don't eat refined sugar. I go to the doctor when I need to. I see the dentist regularly. I bought a WaterPik and use it daily. I do those things because if I'm going to obey what God tells me, then I need to be a good steward of the life he has given me. And that means taking good care of myself in a loving and *effective* manner.

Father, help me to see myself as you see me: loved, valuable, and worth the time and effort it takes to take care of the body you gave me. In Jesus' name, amen.

by Debbie

August 16

See, the Sovereign Lord comes with power . . . He tends his flock like a shepherd: He gathers the lambs in his arms and carries them close to his heart.
Isaiah 40:10–11

I picked up some change from my desk. In it was a quarter stamped with the year 1966, my birth year. It looks like it's been through the ringer. It was darker than the other quarters I was holding. The face was barely visible. I looked at the quarter and thought, *This quarter is old. It looks very rough. But this quarter is still worth twenty-five cents. The value hasn't changed at all. It's still the same.*

Our looks can change. We may have put on extra weight that needs to come off. But our worth is still the same. We haven't depreciated in value because we're older or less beautiful. We haven't changed in God's eyes. He still values us as much as the day he brought us into this world.

A friend of mine put it this way. She said, "We're sheep, right? Well, picture a herd of sheep. They're pretty much the same. There isn't one sheep that's more special to the herder than another. The shepherd takes care of each of the sheep. All of the sheep. When God looks down on us, he sees us as *his* sheep. The ones he loves very much."

How do we look at ourselves? We are still of value. We are still special. So we have some weight to lose. I know people who have some hair to grow (don't tell my husband I said that). Let's see ourselves today as God sees us. Let's quit our stinkin' thinkin' and find the glory in who we are right now!

Lord, you are the Good Shepherd. Thank you for loving me as I am, for rescuing me when I go astray. For caring for me always. In Jesus' name, amen.

by Nancy

August 17

See what great love the Father has lavished on us,
that we should be called children of God!
1 John 3:1

How do we see God? As we do our earthly father? I think a lot of us do. Yet that can warp our perception of who God really is. Some have been abused by their dads, so they see God as abusive and harsh. Some have been judged by their father, so they see God as hard to please. Some don't feel loved or accepted by their father, so they don't feel loved by God.

Yet—when we can see God for who he truly is, freedom will come. I often feel bogged down at my own hands. I feel that I have to be perfect. I have to work to get God to love me. That I have to earn God's love. And try as I might, I just can't do that. And I end up feeling defeated.

That's when I fully realize that God is not a mere human. He is God Almighty. He's given all he has for me. For me! For you! His love is so different from ours. We could never imagine how much love and compassion he has for us. His love is unending. He's not sitting up there in heaven with a stick ready to whack us for every little mistake. He's not up there telling the angels, "Nope, she blew it today, I'm done with her."

Instead, he loves us. He knows our sin and forgives us when we ask. He accepts us the way we are and then works within us to make us better. I need to take time today to find out just how very much my Father in heaven loves me. He loves you! You!

Father, keep me from feeling like a failure, from feeling defeated all the time. Help me be strong enough to conquer this weight issue, in your power. In Jesus' name, amen.

by Nancy

August 18

Have you not known? Have you not heard? The Lord is the everlasting God, the Creator of the ends of the earth. He does not faint or grow weary; his understanding is unsearchable.
Isaiah 40:28 ESV

Who is the God of your understanding? Here's how I see him (in part):

> *My God cares for me as one of his own. He anticipates my needs and meets them, even before I know what they are. He's a guide when I'm lost and a teacher when I need to learn. I can ask him any question. He's patient with me, even when I'm ignorant, unwise, and rebellious.*
>
> *He comforts me when I'm sad and rejoices with me when I'm happy. He holds me when I'm frightened and reassures me that he's there with me.*
>
> *He stands and defends me. He sends his angels to guard and protect me. His nickname for me is "Precious." He gathers me in his arms and touches his forehead to mine.*
>
> *He cares for those I love better than I ever could, often just because I ask him to and because he loves them too.*
>
> *He is building for me my dream home, and one glorious day will take me there to live.*

This is the kind of God I can trust with everything, including with my eating choices, my eating struggles, and my journey toward a healthy body weight.

Father, I know you're so much more that I can ever understand. Help me to see more of who you are every day. In Jesus' name, amen.

by Debbie

August 19

For no one ever hated his own flesh, but nourishes and cherishes it, just as Christ does the church.
Ephesians 5:29 ESV

Therefore, I urge you, brothers and sisters, in view of God's mercy, to offer your bodies as a living sacrifice, holy and pleasing to God—this is your true and proper worship. Do not conform to the pattern of this world, but be transformed by the renewing of your mind. Then you will be able to test and approve what God's will is—his good, pleasing and perfect will.
Romans 12:1–2

My dietician is always telling me that it is time to get selfish. But there are two ways of looking at it. One, it *is* selfish to not think of our families and instead choose the food. Two, *we need to be selfish* by deciding we'll do this for ourselves.

My dietician reminded me that I have put the kids at the forefront of my life for so long that now that they're adults, she wants me to let them go and take care of myself for once. As she said about one of my prodigals, "There's nothing you can do about that. But eating healthy is something you can do for yourself."

So there comes a time when we have to say to the people around us, "You know what? This is important to me, and I'm going to do it. If it means less time dealing with other things, then so be it." Why? Because I'm just as important as my husband and my kids.

Father, thank you for putting someone in my life to remind me that I'm important too. Help me learn to love myself the way that you love me. In Jesus' name, amen.

by Nancy

August 20

We have come to know and have believed the love which God has for us. God is love, and the one who remains in love remains in God, and God remains in him. By this, love is perfected with us, so that we may have confidence in the day of judgment; because as He is, we also are in this world. There is no fear in love, but perfect love drives out fear, because fear involves punishment, and the one who fears is not perfected in love.
1 John 4:16–18

What do I fear? Failure? Success? What others think of me? Do I fear lost friendships when I reach my goal? How I'll look at myself? Do I fear the loss of a food that has been a longtime friend? But the Lord says, "Do not be dismayed. I will strengthen you and help you." But he can't help me if I don't ask, and if I'm not willing.

It's like watching someone I love who's messing up his life. I want to fix him. But he wants no part of it. Even if he did, I can't really fix him. That's how it is with God. He's offering help. He's offering his hand, and how often have I said, "Not yet, Lord, let me try this first." So he allows me to wander a bit more. I'm sure he wishes I would choose to grab his hand.

Then comes the time that I do grab his hand. I begin to trust his love for me. There is no fear in love, but perfect love casts out fear. I know I can't do it on my own. But if I run to the Father as a child does when her daddy gets home from work, he's waiting with open arms. I have so much to tell my Dad.

God, my Father, can I run to you and say, "Do you know what happened today?" Can you help me with my worries, my failures, my sorrows? Can you help me listen to your response? Can you be my Daddy God who loves me? Thank you that I can! In Jesus' name, amen.

by Nancy

August 21

The eyes of the Lord move to and fro throughout the earth that He may strongly support those whose heart is completely His.
2 Chronicles 6:19 NASB

Reading that scripture fills my heart with gratitude. I'm so thankful that God cares enough to search me out, to see all my hard work, to know when I'm really seeking him, trusting him, loving him. I need to know that. I need to know he strongly supports me.

It's significant that every time God gives a promise, he also qualifies it. He promised a land flowing with milk and honey to the Israelites, but they had to forsake their idols. He promised an everlasting kingdom to King David's descendants, *if* they would continually serve him. He loves me, but he wants me to trust him. And he often promised bad things as well—if we don't serve God, if we forsake his ways—there will be consequences.

I've experienced many negative consequences for the time I went my own way as a young adult. Even when I turned back to him as a young mother, I was still forsaking his way when it came to food. And I suffered the consequences for doing that. I was pre-diabetic, had high blood pressure, and the extra weight on my body caused severe osteoarthritis in my knees and back. Now that I've lost some weight, my blood sugar has returned to normal, but the arthritis remains. Yet I've made my peace with that and with God. My sense of his love and presence is profound. He has taken such good care of me, meeting all my physical and spiritual needs. And now, I hope, my heart and my life are completely his, including my food.

Father, thank you for searching for me, even when I was running. In Jesus' name, amen.

by Debbie

August 22

Every good gift and every perfect gift is from above, coming down from the Father of lights with whom there is no variation or shadow due to change.
James 1:17 ESV

People sometimes wonder how, with all my health problems, I can count God as being faithful. Let me count the ways. Even in the darkest times he was right there with me. I've been through hell and back, and I've always known he was right there with me. Even before I really knew him, I somehow knew that he was there. He has never turned his back on me. He has never said, "I give up on you." He kept running after me. Somewhere deep inside, I knew he was calling me. And since I've given my life to him, he has been so faithful.

Sometimes I don't always remember the things he has done, but if I would just take a moment, I can think of many. There have been times of giving and times of comforting. I was so angry with God when I lost my second child, but he didn't step away. Even in that anger I felt him holding me tight.

Now it seems that my fibromyalgia is attacking in different ways. Yet I still feel God with me. I still believe that he's right beside me. And I'm clinging all the harder to him. He's always been faithful and good to me! I'll sing that out until my last breath. Even if the healing never comes. When I die, I'll run to my Father's arms and thank him for everything. God wants to help all of us. He wants to help us through each struggle. He's running after you too. His goodness is there for you. It is there!

Father, I lift up each person reading this. Thank you for all you've given them. You're so faithful and good. I pray blessings over the one reading this now. In Jesus' name, amen!

by Nancy

August 23

This is the day that the Lord has made; let us rejoice and be glad in it.
Psalm 118:24 ESV

They say that laughter is good for the soul. I believe that. When I can find joy in something each day it sure makes my day brighter. I feel better physically. Mentally, I feel on top of the world. It's the opposite if I am having one of those down days. Nothing seems to go right. I feel like I just want to give up. It affects me mentally and physically.

I look around and see all that God has given us. Even on a rainy day I can thank God for giving the land a drink. I like a song where the lyrics say, "I'm thirsty anyway, so bring on the rain."

I can find joy in the simple and the complex. I look around and see the growth of flowers. All the beauty. I look up at the sky and see how it's different every day. I look closely at the snow and see how intricate the flakes are. I'm always amazed at the beauty that surrounds me every day, yet there are some days I just can't see it.

I'm going to make the conscious effort to look for that beauty every day. I'll dance in the rain. I'll see the beauty in the clouds. It sure is better than dwelling on the negative.

Father, help me see the beauty and the joy in each day as I go through this journey of trying to lose weight, of trying to break my addiction. Lord, show me the beauty even in that. Each day means I'm one step closer to victory. One step closer toward my goal. I have one more chance at learning something new. One more chance to look back at how far you've brought me. Thank you, Father, for each little victory. Thank you, Father, for each big victory. And thank you for all the beauty that surrounds me. In Jesus' name, amen.

by Nancy

August 24

You prepare a table before me in the presence of my enemies.
You anoint my head with oil; my cup overflows.
Psalm 23:5

I hadn't paid much attention to this portion of the Twenty-third Psalm until I heard it sung (many years ago now) by Rick Riso on an Integrity Music album about spiritual warfare. I listened closely and suddenly realized how profound these words really are.

I think of King David, perhaps before he took the throne, surrounded by his enemies who were seeking to kill him without cause. God was protecting and providing for him. Samuel had anointed him with oil to proclaim David the new king. David also wrote of a cup filled past the brim as God provided *abundantly* with an overflowing blessing, an overflowing of the Holy Spirit's presence. Right in the midst of his troubles.

As I listened, I felt God say to me, *I'm doing the same for you.* He was fighting for me. Protecting me. Caring for me. Providing for me. Healing me to the point where my cup could overflow.

For most of us, there are areas of our life where we need God to do the fighting for us. Things we need him to heal us from. Things from childhood. From our teens. From our early adult years. Maybe some things that have happened recently or are happening now. Yet if we don't turn to God and ask him to heal our spirits and our minds, we may turn to food instead. After all, it was my comfort for years. Food is fun. Sometimes it was my only friend. And it doesn't let you down like people so often do. Except food can't really heal, can it? God wants us to turn to him for our healing instead, and he's right there, just waiting to bless us until our cup overflows.

Father, thank you for being there to heal my hurting heart. Amen.

by Debbie

August 25

Praise be to the God and Father of our Lord Jesus Christ, who has blessed us in heavenly realms with every spiritual blessing in Christ.
Ephesians 1:3

Sometimes I can get comfortable in the pain. Sometimes I wonder how I would even handle a different life. I have fibromyalgia, and I have often wondered what it would feel like to wake up without pain.

I wonder what would happen if I started with simple praise. If I could change my thinking. Instead of living in the pain and defeat I often feel, what if I thought first to give praise? What can I praise God for? I have so much to be thankful for. The biggest thing for me is that he loves me so much that he's willing to fight for me. He wants me to succeed. He wants me to attain victory. He challenges me to see that too. He challenges me to see what it looks like to succeed.

Most of us at one time or another have lost weight and then gained it back. I once lost almost eighty pounds. I felt so good about myself. I was so happy. Then it came back. Why? Was it because I started concentrating on the negative again?

I used to smoke. When I quit, I read scripture when I wanted a cigarette. Is that something I need to do with food as well? When I want a snack, I could snack on God's word. I need to continue to strive to spend daily time with the Lord. He has so much he wants to share with me. He has such a desire to see me succeed. One of the things I can do is sing a little louder to the Lord—when I do that, I can't put food in my mouth.

Father, help me focus on you and on your word. Take my mind off my troubles and off myself. Make me willing to change. In Jesus' name, amen.

by Nancy

August 26

Because he himself suffered when he was tempted,
he is able to help those who are being tempted.
Hebrews 2:18

For we do not have a high priest who is unable to empathize
with our weaknesses, but we have one who has been tempted
in every way, just as we are—yet he did not sin.
Hebrews 4:15

It's so wonderful to know that we love and serve a God who understands. I never thought about it until I read these scriptures in the book of Hebrews, but if Jesus was tempted in *every* way, then he was tempted with food just like I am. That means he understands me, how my mind and body work—or more precisely, how they don't work correctly—when it comes to food.

Even better, these scriptures tell me that it's exactly because he was tempted like me that he can help me when I'm being tempted. That fills my heart with gratitude. God understands what I'm going through because Jesus experienced it in a physical body that had the same needs as I do. He breathed air; he drank water; he ate food. That means he got thirsty and hungry and had to fulfill those needs. He understands. That's an amazing thing.

Not only were we created in his image, we were created to be in fellowship with God. He knew our need before he ever said, "Let there be light." He had a plan in place before there was an "In the beginning." That shows me the depth of God's love for human beings. The depth of his love for me.

Father, thank you for showing me your love. Thank you for planning things so you'd really know what it's like to be human. In Jesus' name, amen.

by Debbie

August 27

Greater love has no one than this: to lay down one's life for one's friends.
John 15:13

We send invitations to people we want to come to our weddings. We invite people over for a barbecue. We invite people to all sorts of things. We even invite people to our problems when we talk to them about them. But do we take the time to invite God? Do we send him an invitation?

I work at a church, and one day I decided to walk around the building after work. As I walked, I listened to a song that says, "Father can you hear me? I need you now." The thing is—I need God every single day of my life. Even when things are going well, I still need him to celebrate with me. I still need him to protect me. He's my friend. He's my support. And he likes a party just as much as anyone.

Sometimes we see God as this sober-minded being. But he wants to celebrate each milestone with us. He wants to laugh and joke with us. He wants to be our friend in every way, not just be our problem solver. Can we invite him to our barbecues? Can we invite him to celebrate the good decisions we made today?

Sometimes even church can be a challenge—but what if we invited him to church? What if we said, "Lord, I invite you here today. Celebrate with me. Draw me closer to you."? I want to invite God to help me in this weight-loss journey. I want him to walk with me through the challenges—and the celebrations.

Father, I invite you into every aspect of my life. I want you to celebrate with me. To cry with me. I want you to help me. I want to walk with you like I do with my friends. I love you, Lord, with all my heart. I cannot wait to have all my great moments with you. In Jesus' name, amen.

by Nancy

August 28

For no one is cast off by the Lord forever. Though he brings grief, he will show compassion, so great is his unfailing love.
Lamentations 3:31–32

What, then, shall we say in response to these things? If God is for us, who can be against us? He who did not spare his own Son, but gave him up for us all—how will he not also, along with him, graciously give us all things? Who will bring any charge against those whom God has chosen? It is God who justifies. Who then is the one who condemns? No one. Christ Jesus who died—more than that, who was raised to life —is at the right hand of God and is also interceding for us.
Romans 8:31–34

It's such a great comfort to me that God cares for me despite my many failings. Not only that, but in his word he makes specific promises to me as a believer. Though he may discipline me, he also shows me mercy and grace. Though I deserve to be separated from him, he promises to give me good gifts. Though I may deserve condemnation, Jesus chooses not to do that and instead asks God to help me.

The best part is that Jesus knows me. He knows everything about me. It makes me think of how God took care of the prophet Elijah after Jezebel threatened him. Elijah didn't recognize it, but God knew he was exhausted and that he needed rest and food. It makes me think of the talk Jesus had with the Samaritan woman at the well. He saw her; he knew her. God sees me. He knows me. The real me. And he loves me anyway.

Father, thank you for knowing everything about me and loving me anyway. Thank you for all the wonderful plans you have for my life. Amen.

by Debbie

August 29

So God created mankind in his own image, in the image of God he created them; male and female he created them.
Genesis 1:27

The beauty of this world often takes my breath away. My friend is an awesome gardener; she plants beautiful flowers of all different colors and shapes. I look around and see the green grass. Then there's the sky that never looks the same two days in a row. Rainbows are so lovely with all their colors. As I get older, I don't enjoy snow as much, but I even find beauty in that.

I look at things that people have created. Some homes that people build are stunning. Debbie (my fellow author here) is an awesome photographer. I look at her pictures and I'm just in awe at how God really has created a wonderful world for us. There is so much beauty on earth, my list could go on and on.

Do I take time to stop and enjoy it? To think about how intricately God made all these things? How intricately he made you and me? I think he's been trying to tell me something lately. More people have told me how beautiful I am. But I don't take compliments well. I always say thanks, even though I think they can't possibly mean it. I can see beauty in everything else, yet I can't seem to see it in myself. If I could let God show me the beauty in every part of me, just maybe I could beat this weight problem. Maybe I'll see the beauty, inside and out, and want to let it shine. If only I could remind myself that God created me to be unique. That he made me for a purpose. That he wants me to see the beauty of his creation, even in myself!

Father, help me see the beauty in what you created me to be. Help me bring that beauty out in all areas of my life. In Jesus' name, amen.

by Nancy

August 30

And I heard a loud voice from the throne saying, "Look! God's dwelling place is now among the people, and he will dwell with them. They will be his people, and God himself will be with them and be their God. 'He will wipe every tear from their eyes. There will be no more death' or mourning or crying or pain, for the old order of things has passed away."
Revelation 21:3–4

This isn't the first time in scripture that we see God's encouragement about how things will ultimately turn out for his people (see Isaiah 25:8). I've been rereading the *Left Behind* series; I know that things are unlikely to turn out exactly as portrayed in the novels, but they're encouraging just the same. And I know the authors have a few things right. One of them is their portrayal of God's grace and mercy in the midst of end-times judgments. Another is how much God loves us, including those whose hearts are still in rebellion. And how much he knows and loves *me.*

Knowledge of God's love helps me keep going when I'm weary and weak. His love reminds me when I've strayed, and it's his gentle tugging in my spirit that puts me back on the right path. He cares about every aspect of my life. My worries, my hopes, my dreams, my family, my regrets, and my future. He cares about my weight. He knows how many hairs I have on my head, which means he knows me better than I know myself. When he asks me to change something about my diet, that means I can trust him to know what's best for me. I love God. But only because he first loved me. His love is so big, it's overwhelming. But knowing he loves me fills me with gratitude. His love changes everything.

Father, thank you for your great love for me. It gives me such strength and hope. It's what makes me love you in return. All praise to you! Amen.

by Debbie

August 31

But by the grace of God I am what I am, and his grace to me was not without effect. No, I worked harder than all of them—yet not I, but the grace of God that was with me.
1 Corinthians 15:10

Grace is defined both as "unmerited favor" and "to be courteous." Do I have grace toward myself? How many times do I show grace to other people? How often am I courteous to those around me? Then I turn on myself. I don't show myself the same favor. I need to change that. Someone once told me that whatever I can't say to a friend or to my child, I'd better not say to myself. I would never think to call anyone some of the things I've called myself. If I could just put that rule in effect in my life, just maybe that grace would help lift me out of the mire and bring me toward the road to freedom. To peace of mind. To victory.

Jesus laid down his life that we would be set free. That truly is amazing grace. The chaos in our lives can be set free by his grace. Can I accept it for myself? Can I accept his unfailing love? I believe anyone can. I believe we can be set free. We can be ourselves. We can walk with a smile on our face because we've been set free. We've shown ourselves grace.

It makes me excited to think that we can walk in total freedom. Do you all feel like yelling it out, like me? We can be who we're meant to be! We can walk each day in freedom! Whew! I'll take it, Lord! Just sprinkle a little grace over our lives today, tomorrow, and always.

Father, help me see that I need to show myself grace. I need to be courteous to myself. I need to step into your amazing grace and taste the freedom. Oh, Lord, how light I'll feel! Pour it on, please, Lord! In Jesus name, amen.

by Nancy

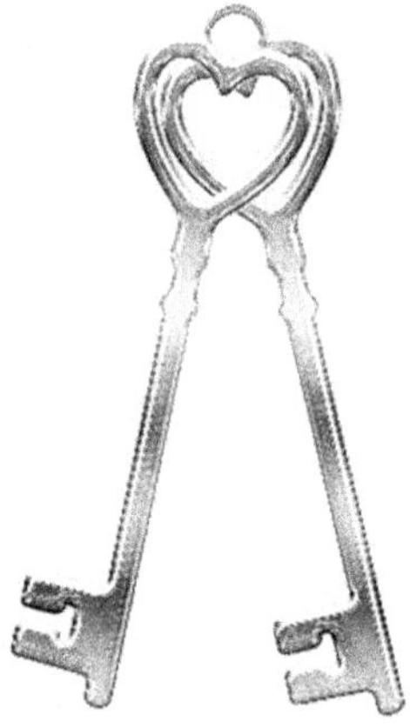

RESPONSIBILITY

We work to make things right with people and with God.

Cry of Our Hearts

September 1

But each person is tempted when he is lured and enticed by his own desire.
James 1:14

So I say, walk by the Spirit, and you will not gratify the desires of the flesh.
Galatians 5:16

In my weight-loss journey, I finally began to understand that I was running from my own unhappiness. Running straight to food. Then I began to understand that there was a way out. Just like the Lord made a way out of sin through his sacrifice, just like eternal life is a gift, freedom from the compulsion to overeat can also be a gift. But first I have to admit that I cannot do it myself. I have to turn my will and my life (regarding food) over to him. To keep the compulsion from returning, I have to confess my sins and deal with the emotions and other aspects of my life that are pushing me to the food.

Sometimes I eat because I'm bored. Other times because I'm frustrated about something. Or fearful. Or resentful. Or angry. Maybe I haven't forgiven someone I need to forgive. Or maybe I'm feeling guilty about something I did that I shouldn't have done. Maybe I'm the one who needs to ask for forgiveness. Maybe I need to pay restitution for something I damaged or stole, even if it was long ago. Whatever it is, I need to make it right. Only then am I ready to accept the gift that God so wants to give me—the ability to eat in a healthy way.

Father, show me what's really bothering me, and when I finally see, help me to do what I need to do to make it right again. In Jesus' name, amen.

by Debbie

September 2

Every good and perfect gift is from above, coming down from the Father of the heavenly lights, who does not change like shifting shadows.
James 1:17

Everything we have comes from God. If we own a house, we can follow the path backward, and we see it all begins with God. He took care of us through childhood. Then we became adults, and he provided a job. That job meant we had the money to buy a house. He led us to where he wanted us and to the house that met our needs.

Every decision we make impacts so many other decisions. I have a daughter who was in a snowmobile accident. I've often wondered if we had chosen not to move to our current home, would she have been in the place where she could get hurt? Sometimes we take our decisions so callously that we don't think about how they may impact the people around us and what may happen in coming years. The best way to handle it is to give it all to God. As horrible as our daughter's accident was, in some ways it was a blessing, because it also saved her from some choices she had been making.

It's the same with eating. Each decision we make with our food impacts our life in some way or another, either for better or for worse. But I do know that God wants to guide us in our decisions. And he wants to reward us with good things. Many times I think I can reward myself, but he can give me much greater rewards that I can ever imagine. My job is simply to talk to him and trust him.

Father, make me willing to listen to your quiet guidance. I so look forward to the rewards you have in store for me. In Jesus name, amen.

by Nancy

September 3

And do not lead us into temptation, but deliver us from evil.
Matthew 6:13

I was reading Carol Kent's *A New Kind of Normal.* In the book, a woman described how she had the perfect marriage. They were really happy. The kids were happy. They did well in school. They were always laughing and joking. She and her husband went on romantic getaways.

Then the oldest moved out to attend college. Then the next one. She noticed that her husband had withdrawn and was not as jovial as usual. One night she went to talk to him about it and she discovered he had been viewing pornography since before they were married. They each saw counselors, and he promised he would never do it again. But he did do it again. Repeatedly.

Then their oldest child became addicted to drugs and spent eighteen months in jail. Another child became an alcoholic and went in and out of rehab. The youngest felt like he had to be "the perfect one," which caused him to battle depression.

What got my attention was that they realized that addictions are passed down through generations. Until someone breaks the cycle. They decided that her husband had to come clean to the children. Their hope is that they'll be the last generation to battle with addiction. If your addiction is food, are you willing to be the generation where the addiction is broken so that you don't pass it along to your children? The only way to do that is to turn to the Lord for the strength that you don't have to overcome it.

Father, help me to break the pattern of addiction in my family. Help me take responsibility for starting the change. And again, I ask, please help me. In Jesus' name, amen.

by Nancy

September 4

Do not take revenge, my dear friends, but leave room for God's wrath, for it is written: "It is mine to avenge; I will repay," says the Lord.
Romans 12:19

If you've lived long enough, there has already come a time, and probably several times, when people have done something really wrong to you. They've wounded you. Physically. Financially. Emotionally. They've broken your trust. Betrayed you. It's been to the point where you've wanted to get back at those people. You wanted justice. Maybe even to hurt them in the way they hurt you.

Scripture is quite clear on this subject. We are to leave recompense in God's hands. Justice is his, not ours. And we are to pray for our enemies. For those who persecute us. For those who hurt us, no matter in what way they have done so.

This is one of the most difficult aspects of the Christian message. It doesn't mean we can't acknowledge our feelings of wanting revenge. Wanting justice and desiring the people who have hurt us to understand exactly what they've done—that's natural. It's how we choose to act upon those feelings that is vital to our own well-being.

I can't carry out my own revenge, and I can't let bitterness take root, because if I do I'll inevitably turn to food to comfort me. I have to deal with those feelings as soon as they arise and give them—and the person who hurt me—to God to deal with. This is a matter of obedience, but it works in my favor if I do it the way God wants me to. Because letting go makes *me* free.

Father, when I'm hurting, please be my comfort. Let me not give into the desire to make things right on my own. Help me to let it go. In Jesus' name, amen.

by Debbie

September 5

"Woe to the obstinate children," declares the Lord, "to those who carry out plans that are not mine, forming an alliance, but not by my Spirit, heaping sin upon sin."
Isaiah 30:1

"Why do you call me, 'Lord, Lord,' and do not do what I say?"
Luke 6:46

How many of us are living in rebellion? In stubbornness? We don't want to give up the soda pop. We don't want to give up the candy. What do you mean I can't have seconds on Thanksgiving?

We want to cling to the very thing that is killing us physically and spiritually. We tend to not want to think of it as such a bad thing. But sometimes we have to call things as they are: Sin. Rebellion. Stubbornness.

God talks forcefully about these sins, because he knows how much harm they can do to us. How much danger that they put us in. He is our Father. He's trying to protect us from harm, and we just keep stepping right back into that danger. I must be honest with myself. I can't fool myself any longer—my rebellion is killing me one way or another.

But there is hope. If I just turn to him. Then the next step is to repent. Tell him how sorry I am. Make a good effort to step away from the very things that are hurting me. God will help me do that.

How much time are we willing to spend with him to get his help to stop walking in our rebellion?

Lord, you are Lord. Let me begin to act like you are. Help me to take responsibility for my actions so that I'll stop rebelling against you. In Jesus' name, amen.

by Nancy

September 6

My sheep hear my voice, and I know them, and they follow me.
John 10:27

A friend told me about a sermon he heard titled *Are You a Fan or a Follower of Jesus?* For days those words went off in my head. Fan or follower? When I think of a fan, I think of someone at a concert. You like the band. You're excited, so you hoot n' holler. You may even dance. You may be so deep into the music that you lose all sense of time. Yet—has the band brought anything to your world besides a song? Will they help you personally if you're going through a rough time?

We all need a different type of relationship.

In other words, I don't just want to say, "Man, Jesus is cool. I kinda like that he's there whenever I need him." I don't want a one-sided relationship. I don't want to just go to church on Sunday because that's what fans do. I want to go because I'm a follower of Christ. I want to follow him wherever he wants me to go. I want a relationship. I want it for many reasons. First of all, he's my Creator. He's my Father. But he's also my Comforter, my Friend, my Help, my Life.

So what does it mean to be a follower of Christ? I wonder if I followed him in all aspects of my life would I still have weight issues? I tend to eat out of boredom and stress. What if I filled that boredom with the Lord? What if I gave that stress to the Lord? How different could life be?

Father, I want to be your follower, not just your fan. I want to have a relationship with you as my God, as my Savior, and as my friend. Let me take responsibility for my choices—help me choose to follow you. In Jesus' name, amen.

by Nancy

September 7

Have I not commanded you? Be strong and courageous. Do not be terrified; do not be discouraged, for the Lord your God will be with you wherever you go. Go through the camp and tell the people, "Get your supplies ready. Three days from now you will cross the Jordan here to go in and take possession of the land the Lord your God is giving you for your own."
Joshua 1:9,11

Sometimes God speaks in unexpected ways. I was reading the book of Joshua, and the Lord said to me through that scripture that when it comes to my compulsive eating addiction, that I needed to do the same thing that the Israelites did when they were finally ready to go into their "land of milk and honey."

The land that would ultimately become Israel wasn't empty when they entered it. They had to work at taking it; they had to conquer the people in the fortified cities. Yet God said that if they did as he commanded through Moses and Joshua, God would be with them wherever they went, that he would give them victory in the land, that they would take possession of it, that it would be theirs. It's not a coincidence that the name Jesus is actually *Joshua* (*Yeshua* in Hebrew), meaning "salvation."

God was telling me that I needed to conquer my compulsive eating in the same way. He wasn't going to just let me walk into an empty land—there were things there already occupying it that I needed to deal with first: emotions, resentments, unconfessed sins, and more. Not only did I need to clean those things out, but I had to be obedient in trying a different way of eating. I had to take action.

Father, help me to get my supplies ready so that I can follow Yeshua into my own promised land. In Jesus' name, amen.

by Debbie

September 8

Hear my prayer, Lord, listen to my cry for help;
do not be deaf to my weeping.
Psalm 39:12

I was curious how many times the Bible tells us to pray. My research strictly on variations of the word "prayer" shows, according to the *NIV Exhaustive Bible Concordance*, that the word "pray" is used 121 times, "prayed" 68 times, "prayer" 106 times, "prayers" 32 times, "praying" 36 times, and "prays" 12 times, for a total of 375 times. That's how important it is to God that we pray. That we spend time with him.

Sometimes I go to God and ask him once or twice for something and expect a magical solution. I think, well, I *asked*, so now he'll answer. But what if he wants to show us something about what we asked? What if he wants to teach us something through that situation so it doesn't happen again? What if he wants to guide us to a solution?

There have been times that I've asked for a financial blessing, went about my business, and then wondered why I didn't get it. Maybe God wanted to show me how to accomplish it. Maybe he wants me to learn something from the struggle. But I didn't give him the chance. How many times have I asked the Lord to deliver me from obesity. I prayed—and then grabbed a candy bar. Prayer is just the beginning. I also need to listen. Take the time to see what he wants me to do. Maybe he'll tell me to do something. Maybe he'll tell me to rest and let him do the work. Either way, I need to hear it from him.

Father, help me take responsibility for doing more than just asking, for listening to what you want from me. In Jesus' name, amen.

by Nancy

September 9

Jacob replied, "First sell me your birthright." — "Look, I am about to die," Esau said. "What good is the birthright to me?" But Jacob said, "Swear to me first." So he swore an oath to him, selling his birthright to Jacob. Then Jacob gave Esau some bread and some lentil stew. He ate and drank, and then got up and left. So Esau despised his birthright.
Genesis 25:31–34

I was doing my Bible reading one day and came across this scripture. It really got me to thinking. First Esau said that he was starving. I'm thinking he was being a drama king there. I don't believe he would have starved to death. Plus, he could have found something to eat on his own. He just plain wanted the stew.

He *wanted.* He went after what he *wanted.* How many times have I acted based on what I wanted rather than on what I needed? Then he traded his rights as firstborn for the stew. So I started asking myself, what have I traded for that candy bar? What have I traded for that fast food? What am I trading on a daily basis for what God would rather I have instead—good health. Which is good living. Guilt free living. Peace and joy.

What am I trading? If I'm going to be honest, I'm trading everything. Being able to do things with my family. I'm probably trading what I *want* for a shorter life if I don't get this eating problem in line.

Father, you know I'm being irresponsible. You know that I'm rebelling against what I know I should do because of what I want to do. And because of my rebellion, I'm trading what's good for what's temporary. A taste of stew for my very health and well-being. Lord, I've been so foolish! Make me wiser today. Help me make right choices instead of foolish ones, starting today. In Jesus' name, amen.

by Nancy

September 10

Finish each day and be done with it. You have done what you could; some blunders and absurdities have crept in; forget them as soon as you can. Tomorrow is a new day; you shall begin it serenely and with too high a spirit to be encumbered with your old nonsense.
Ralph Waldo Emerson

But one thing I do: Forgetting what is behind and straining toward what is ahead, I press on toward the goal to win the prize for which God has called me heavenward in Christ Jesus.
Philippians 3:13–14

Not only do I need to start each day with prayer and meditation, I need to end it that way as well. I typically spend five minutes reading and a few minutes praying. It helps to review the day to check in with myself and God to see whether I did anything that I need to confess and ask forgiveness for, either from God or from someone else.

It's also important to leave behind those things I've confessed. Once I'm forgiven, I'm forgiven. If God can "forget" my sins, then who am I to hold onto them?

I also need to leave my problems in God's hands. He can take care of even the big problems I'm going through, which means I don't have to do anything about them, because He will, one way or another. Here's a saying I like to remember when I'm facing a situation where I'm completely powerless: I can't, God can, so let him.

Father, help me to take responsibility for what I've done when I should and to forgive myself when I need to, just as you forgive me. Help me to turn my problems over to the only One who can solve them: You. In Jesus' name, amen.

by Debbie

September 11

But we have this treasure in jars of clay to show that this all-surpassing power is from God and not from us.
2 Corinthians 4:7

What is your passion? I heard that question one day. I had to think really hard on it. Do I have a passion? Do I know how to have passion?

What am I truly passionate about in life? At the time, I honestly didn't know that I had ever felt total passion toward anything. Could it be because if I felt passion, chances are I could fail at it? So why stretch myself out there if I have a sense of failure that comes over me?

God was very passionate. He was very passionate for me. He sent His only Son to die for me. Now that is being passionate about something.

God is passionate about wanting me to be healthy. God is passionate about wanting me to be full of joy. God is passionate about helping me do what I need to do to succeed. So if he's that passionate, and his word never fails, then how can I fail?

When I stick with God, all things come together. Failure is not an option.

So I need to search myself to see what I'm passionate about. And I hope that I'll discover that I'm passionate about getting the extra weight off. Because I must remember that I will not fail with God!

Father, please show me my part, my responsibility in success and failure. Help me to be passionate about doing what you want me to do. Help me to turn my life over to you, understanding that you will never let me down. In Jesus' name, amen.

by Nancy

September 12

How often they provoked Him in the wilderness and grieved Him in the desert! Yes, again and again they tempted God and limited the Holy One of Israel.
Psalm 78:40–41

God has been talking to me the last few months about forgiveness. My big thing has always, always been: Why should God bless me when I have made the mistakes?

I'm the one who put the extra food in my mouth. So why should he now help me lose the weight? Think about it this way: If your kids screw up with something, you wouldn't feed them that night? You wouldn't let them sleep in their beds? You'd put them out in the street? Of course not! We all make mistakes.

God has been telling me that I'm the only one holding my mistakes over my head. I'm the only one choosing this way of life as a punishment for the mistakes I've made. That's some pretty stinkin' thinkin' that I need to get rid of.

Yet he forgave me the day I asked him to. He forgot about my sin—my mistake—that very day. He would never withhold something from me because of something I did three months ago. Am I better than him that I could forgive my kids more easily than he can forgive me?

But I tend to think, *How could you forgive me yet again, Lord? I just never change!* In that way I limit God. Yet his forgiveness goes on and on. His mercy is new each morning.

Father, open my eyes to see the true extent of your love, your kindness, and your mercy toward me. Help me to forgive myself in the same way that you have forgiven me. Don't let me get away with limiting your forgiveness. In Jesus' name, amen.

by Nancy

September 13

You shall have no other gods before Me.
Exodus 20:3

Before I gave up sugar, I was afraid to do it. Although I didn't realize it, that's what I relied on to get me through the day. It scared me to think about not ever eating sweets again. It was my comfort.

I tried on my own willpower to give up sugar and white flour, and I messed up for two days straight. But once I started praying and writing and holding myself accountable to another human being and to God for what I put in my mouth, then I could give up the foods I had relied on for so long.

It didn't hurt, and it wasn't as hard as I expected. When I gave up something that had become an idol instead of God, I found that the Lord dealt with me immediately on some things I hadn't wanted to face. And he waited on others. I certainly felt my feelings, and it wasn't always fun. But I had someone to call, I prayed, and I wrote about it, and that allowed me to get through without turning to the foods that caused me to stuff my feelings.

I've been sugar free now for two years. I can do it if I look at it one day at a time. Sometimes it's one meal at a time. Sometimes it's just one urge to eat that I need to get through for five minutes, and then it's gone. It doesn't come naturally to me to wait it out. I even have to work at remembering to turn to God to help me through the feelings, because I've been relying on food for so long to get through them instead. But it works—IF I work at it.

Father, remind me to turn to you when I think I'm hungry but I'm really not. When I think I can't live without something, remind me that it's you that I can't live without. In Jesus' name, amen.

by Debbie

September 14

So David triumphed over the Philistine with a sling and a stone; without a sword in his hand he struck down the Philistine and killed him.
1 Samuel 17:50

Is there anyone in this world who can be my hero? We have such high hopes of our husband or a friend being that person in our lives. But no human can be on a pedestal without feeling the pressure. Firefighters are heroes. Though they may be able to get me out of a burning house, can they keep the structure from being damaged in the fire? We tend to expect a lot out of people. I've said to myself that if I could just get more support, I would lose the weight. But many of my friends *have* offered their support.

I'm sure you're thinking that I'll say that God is our hero. That's a given. But I really want to say that we need to be our own hero. We need to put out that fire inside that wants to destroy us. We need to want to do that. We need to stand up straight. Shake ourselves off and give ourselves a pep talk. We need to tell ourselves "I'll do it." I'll do what needs to be done. I'll be my own hero. I'll stop the self-sabotage. I can succeed. Make sure to stand straight as you tell yourself that. No slumping.

It's time to lift myself up. Between God and me, we've got this. I'm a mighty warrior with the will to do what I need to do. I'll slingshot that enemy right out of my life. Because of God, I'm strong. I'll have what I need. No more excuses. I need to grab the strength I need and run with it. God has already given it to me.

Father, thank you so much for giving me all that I need. Help me stand tall and work with all that you have given me to defeat this giant in my life. Before long that giant will be an ant. In Jesus' precious name, amen.

by Nancy

September 15

My son, if you receive my words and treasure up my commandments with you, making your ear attentive to wisdom and inclining your heart to understanding; yes, if you call out for insight and raise your voice for understanding, if you seek it like silver and search for it as for hidden treasures, then you will understand the fear of the Lord and find the knowledge of God.
Proverbs 2:1–5 ESV

The last couple weeks have been crazy. I've been running non-stop and haven't felt well—because I haven't been taking care of myself. There are things I need to do to maintain my body. I need to eat healthy and rest. Instead, I just plain wore myself down. I put out my lower back and didn't even take the time to notice! Because I have a chronic illness I have to be in tune with my body, because I'm so used to pain that I don't always notice when something is really wrong. This time I had some pinched nerves that caused a great deal of discomfort. It made me realize that I'm not invincible. I need to take better care of myself. I need to follow God's instructions about how to do that. He tells us rest is necessary. He tells us dancing is good. He even tells us what kinds of food to eat if we look closely enough. We just have to slow down enough to look and listen.

I pray that as I grow in the understanding of what God is wanting to share with me that I will first be willing to hear it and then that I will *desire* to hear it.

Father, help me to slow down and learn from you. Help me "hear" what my body is telling me I need at the moment. Help me choose a glass of water instead of a piece of chocolate. Help me be intuitive about what I really have time for and not just jump right in. In Jesus' name, amen.

by Nancy

September 16

For who were those who heard and yet rebelled? Was it not all those who left Egypt led by Moses? And with whom was he provoked for forty years? Was it not with those who sinned, whose bodies fell in the wilderness? And to whom did he swear that they would not enter his rest, but to those who were disobedient? So we see that they were unable to enter because of unbelief.
Hebrews 3:16–18

The Israelites had just come out of Egypt where they had seen a series of miracles that they were appropriately awed by. Yet within days they were already in rebellion. How quickly they turned to idolatry! The Israelites are a perfect illustration of how it isn't just people who are part of the "world" (as the Bible puts it) who rebel. We, even as believers, do it too.

I was just as guilty of idolatry and rebellion—with food. I lived a Christian life in other ways. I went to church, taught Sunday school, helped with Vacation Bible School, and studied the Bible. But every day I also practiced gluttony. Not a pretty word, but it's not a pretty thing. Essentially, I made food more important than God. I paid severe consequences for my rebellion. My blood pressure climbed high enough to require medication, my blood sugar reached the prediabetic range, and the extra weight took its toll on my knees, causing osteoarthritis, which effectively disabled me. I still walk with a severe limp.

There is a way out. God calls us to put him first, but he doesn't require us to use our own strength to overcome our weakness. We do have to make a choice, though, to take certain actions that will lead us on the road to recovery.

Father, let me always remember to put no other gods before you. Amen.

by Debbie

September 17

Jesus asked him, "Judas, are you betraying the Son of Man with a kiss?"
Luke 22:48

I've caught myself being very judgmental of my extended family. I've sometimes said to myself, *Well that's just horrible. I don't know if I can forgive that. How could a good Christian do something like that? Are they even a Christian?*

Then I got a wake-up "slap" from God. My eyes were opened to the idea that he sees no sin worse than another. So—my sins of gluttony, greed for food, and all the others that go with overeating need to be seen as they are. Sin!

But has it become such a norm for me that I'm not walking daily in repentance? Each day, have I repented for the extra things I ate that I didn't need? Have I repented for not choosing the healthier option? Have I repented for not taking care of this temple of the Holy Spirit? Or has my sin just become normal to me? Understanding that truth brings tears to my eyes. It's so easy to think, *Oh, their sin is much worse than what I'm doing.* But it's not.

In the drama *The Living Last Supper*, the narrator introduces each person at the table, then talks about the betrayal of Jesus. Each person at the table then asks, "Is it me? Is it me?"

Is it me? Am I betraying Jesus daily in my eating? I answer that question with tears in my eyes: "Yes, it is me." Yes, I have betrayed him in many areas of my life. Yet all he desires is for me to be healthy.

Is it me, Lord? Is it me?

Father, I repent of all my wrongdoing. I repent of my betrayal. I repent of my gluttony. I repent of my rebellion and selfishness. Turn my heart back toward you, Lord, and give me the power to do the right thing. In Jesus' name, amen.

by Nancy

September 18

Where there is no guidance, a people falls,
but in an abundance of counselors there is safety.
Proverbs 11:14 ESV

Above all else, guard your heart, for everything you do flows from it.
Let your eyes look straight ahead; fix your gaze directly before you.
Proverbs 4:23, 25

There are so many scriptures that tell us to be careful who we hang out with. I know for me it's very important. If I'm around negative people a lot, then I tend to lean that way. If I'm around angry people, then I tend to find things to be angry about. Or I become frustrated.

But if I'm around encouraging people, people who laugh and look for the blessings in life, then I do that too.

I have even found the same thing is true of what I watch on TV. If I watch a show where everyone is always mad, it brings me down. Yet if I watch a comedy or an uplifting movie, then my life, my feelings, seem to be balanced.

God talks about being careful what we put in our minds. I really believe he knew that he had to say that because of the times we're living in. Times when we are constantly bombarded by images and messages in the media, many of which do not honor God.

Father, I pray that you would help me to surround myself with encouragers, with people who appreciate all you do for them. Lord, may I also be that for others. I pray that I will be an encourager and good counsel to others. Lord, may I be responsible with my words, so that your light will shine through me every day. In Jesus' name, amen.

by Nancy

September 19

You, therefore, have no excuse, you who pass judgment on someone else, for at whatever point you judge another, you are condemning yourself, because you who pass judgment do the same things.
Romans 2:1

One of my least favorite aspects of human nature is the tendency to blame someone else for our own failings. Have you ever been on the receiving end of that blame? I have, and it's not fun—you realize pretty quickly that you've been blamed for something over which you actually have no control whatsoever.

We've all done it in one way or another. It's one of the first things humans did in the Garden of Eden after eating the forbidden fruit: Adam blamed Eve. Eve blamed the snake.

Blaming someone for our failings is a huge part of addictive behavior. As someone who has struggled with overeating most of my life, at different times I have blamed others (if he would only not bring home those donuts!), my circumstances (I'm working so many hours, I just don't have time), others again (my coworkers bring in so many goodies that I can't resist!), my genetics (thanks a lot, DNA!), or my upbringing (Mom cooked like a good Midwesterner—so I grew up eating lots of meat, potatoes, fast food, and gooey homemade desserts) *ad infinitum.*

It's only when I stop blaming and take responsibility for my own choices, for my own actions, that I can finally live in recovery. It's only then that I can begin to take the right actions that will see me onto the path toward victorious living.

Father, keep me from blaming other people for my own failings. Help me to take responsibility for what I've done and for my own decisions and actions. In Jesus' name, amen.

by Debbie

September 20

A certain man was preparing a great banquet and invited many guests.
At the time of the banquet he sent his servant to tell those
who had been invited, "Come, for everything is now ready."
But they all alike began to make excuses.
Luke 14:16–18

Seems to me I always throw diets to the wind on the weekends. Or when my stress level is up. I would love to blame it on my husband or kids: "They caused me to stress out, so I ate." But it all comes down to ME. It's my job to learn how to deal with the stress.

I was singing during worship one Sunday and realized I don't want to just do lip service to my King. The song said, "Take my heart and transform it, take my mind and conform it." I wondered, *Do I really want you to change my heart and mind, Lord? Do I really want You to take this sin from me?* I believe the answer is yes, but how badly do I want it? Enough to lay the stuff aside that I would love to shove in my mouth?

God says his word is my bread. So why do I have to shove more actual bread down my throat? I'm not saying to not eat at all. But I am saying cut back. Say no to some of it. Would I still be alive at noon if I only had one slice of toast in the morning?

I'm going to cut back this week and see if I'm still alive next week. I'll tell my friends and family to stay tuned. They may hear my tummy growl, but this is a test, and only a test, of my stomach's broadcast system. All joking aside, it's time to take the weekends—and the stress—by storm.

Father, give me the strength to do what I can't do on my own power—to do your will when it comes to food. In Jesus' name, amen.

by Nancy

September 21

Do you see a man who is hasty in his words?
There is more hope for a fool than for him.
Proverbs 29:20 ESV

One thing God has shown me is about my reactions. How do I react to situations? Do I try to find the positive? Or do I go straight to the negative?

The other morning, I got up and something happened. At this writing I can't even remember what it was! Some tiny thing. At the time, I remember thinking to myself, *Oh, great. This is how today is going to go. Guess this will be a bad day*. It was the simplest thing, yet I made it so big that I was ready to let it ruin my whole day.

When someone in the car ahead of me does something dumb, my hasty words come out pretty quickly. As I stand at the checkout stand at the grocery store and I'm thinking how horrible this day has been, suddenly there's a candy bar just screaming out to me. After all, I "deserve" it after putting up with what has happened all day, right? No, no, NO! God says, "There is more hope for a fool" than for someone who speaks in haste.

I wonder what would happen if I took time to calm my mind. Stop and think first. Take a PAUSE. Better yet—stop and ask God for help. If I did those things before I take a negative action, before I react, how would my day go then? How would my life go?

Father, I pray that my mouth will not speak out of haste. I pray that my heart will not react in haste. Please calm my mind and help me to focus on you. Lord, may my mouth and my mind line up with your words. In Jesus' name, amen.

by Nancy

September 22

I find space for what I treasure, I make time for what I want
I choose my priorities and Jesus you're my number one
So I will make room for you, I will prepare for two
So you don't feel that you can't live here, please live in me
My will (You can move that over)
My way (You can move that over)
My ego (You can move that over)
My plans (You can move that over)
From Make Room, *a song by Jonathan McReynolds*

Riches I heed not, nor man's empty praise,
Thou mine inheritance, now and always
Thou, and Thou only, first in my heart,
High King of Heaven, my treasure Thou art
From the traditional hymn, Be Thou My Vision

We live in a culture in which, arguably, many of us have more leisure time than people had at any other time in history. That means we can spend a good chunk of our time exactly how we choose. Recently, what I do with my time has changed considerably. I have added daily actions that contribute significantly to my recovery from compulsive eating. A typical day means prayer and reading scriptures and recovery literature upon awakening and more reading and praying at bedtime. These actions have become habits essential to maintaining my recovery from compulsive eating and the resulting weight loss. The truth is that I spend my precious time on what I treasure. That's why I spend time every day working to maintain my recovery.

Father, never let me forget to treasure you with my time. In Jesus' name, amen.

by Debbie

September 23

And he said to them, "Come away by yourselves to a desolate place and rest a while." For many were coming and going, and they had no leisure even to eat.
Mark 6:31

It's so easy for me to want to do for everyone else. I have work to do. I have cleaning to do. I have to take care of everyone. So where do I fall in all this "doing"? At the end of the line. I end up growing weary at the end of the day, and the rest of my life seems overwhelming. Jesus tells us that we need rest. There are times when we need to just "be."

Do I take the time each day for that? There are a few people in my life whom I admire. They get up early every day so they can have quiet time. One works out, and the other has a prayer time.

When I think of getting up early, it's so hard for me to even consider. Yet I think that my day would go so much better if I were not so rushed in the mornings. By taking care of myself and making time, I would have time to myself. If I did that, not only would I grow mentally and spiritually, but I would also benefit physically.

I need to find a time that will work for me. A time when I have energy. Putting it off till the end of the day won't work if I'm so weary that I can't focus enough to just "be" with God.

Father, please show me when you want me to make time for you. Time that I can use to just rest in you. Time when I should be taking the rest that I need for my body as well as my mind. I pray, then, that it will become a habit that I would miss if I didn't do it. Thank you, Lord, for showing me through your word what I need to do to be whole. In Jesus' name, amen.

by Nancy

September 24

So do not throw away your confidence; it will be richly rewarded. You need to persevere so that when you have done the will of God, you will receive what he has promised.
Hebrews 10:35–36

What has God promised me? Direction, help, wisdom, peace, joy, strength, sustenance, deliverance from temptation, healing, and restoration. He has promised much more, but those are the things I think of as I walk on this path to weight loss.

As is true with almost all of God's promises, there are conditions. These often fall into the categories of belief, confession, obedience, and perseverance.

There's give and take in all relationships. It's a partnership involving free will on both sides. My relationship with God is no different. Though it's unequal (he's eternal and all-powerful; I'm weak and mortal), he is willing to provide everything I need. *If* I'm faithful to do the few things that he asks.

On this weight-loss journey, he promises that I will have success. *If*. *If* I pray and ask for his guidance. And once I discover what he wants me to do, then he'll help me *if* I actually follow through. *If* I take action.

If I'm tempted, do I pray first or do I reach for what I want first? Do I make an effort to ask God what he wants me to eat? And how much? And once he tells me, do I say, "Okay, God. I'll do it"? My journey has been one where I've wavered back and forth. When I listen and obey, I succeed. When I go my own way, I don't. I'm grateful I've said "Yes, Lord" more than not.

Father, help me to DO what you've asked me to do. Every time. In Jesus' name, amen.

by Debbie

September 25

Whoever conceals his transgressions will not prosper,
but he who confesses and forsakes them will obtain mercy.
Proverbs 28:13 ESV

I looked up the meaning of being responsible: *being the primary cause of something and so able to be blamed or credited for it.*

Remember when our parents would ask, "Who did this?" No one wanted to step up and take the blame. Or the excuses would start flying. It can be that way with being overweight. Sometimes we want to blame others: "They cause me stress." Or, "He brought donuts home." Sometimes we want to blame life: "If my life were easier." But in the end, it all comes right back to me. I'm the one making the choices. I'm the one doing things that I shouldn't be doing. I'm the one eating the things I should not.

Once we accept responsibility, we realize that it's up to us. It's my decision whether or not to eat those donuts that came home. It's my choice whether the actions of others will make me shove food in my mouth or instead find a better way of dealing with the situation. I'm fully responsible for every choice I make in this life.

Sometimes we want people to pooh-pooh the situation. We want people to say, "Oh, I understand. It's hard to lose when . . . ." But we don't need people to make us feel better. We need people to hold us accountable. To encourage us along the way. There are so many support groups . . . in-person and online. There's no excuse.

So, no more blaming people. It's time to tell God how sorry I am. It's time to be accountable to him and to a friend. And it's time to watch the weight fall off.

Father, help me to make wiser choices. Help me to surround myself with people who love me enough to tell me the truth. In Jesus' name, amen.

by Nancy

September 26

But each person is tempted when he is lured and enticed by his own desire.
James 1:14

The crucible for silver and the furnace for gold, but the Lord tests the heart.
Proverbs 17:3

Scripture assumes that we will be tempted. Just because we come to faith in Christ does not mean we'll suddenly be free from the desire to do what is wrong. The difference is that though we still are tempted, we have a Savior who can provide the means and the strength to overcome it. He puts his Holy Spirit within us at the moment we're born again, and that means we now have power within us too.

But I have to choose to walk in that power. I have to choose to ask God for help when I'm tempted. I have to take responsibility. The truth is that when I give into temptation, it's because I want to. I have a desire, and so I give in. Is it because I'm weak and human? Sometimes. Most often, it's because I'm willful and rebellious. I don't want to do it God's way. I haven't come to the point where I truly believe he knows best.

I believe sometimes God leaves us with our weak spots because he's testing us. He wants to know that we have truly given ourselves wholly to him. The question is: Am I willing to give him every part of me? Including what I choose to eat? The truth is that sometimes I am and sometimes I'm not. But I know that when I say yes to everything he wants, that's when I succeed.

Father, please make me willing to take responsibility for all my actions and to follow you completely, doing everything you ask of me. In Jesus' name, amen.

by Debbie

September 27

Therefore confess your sins to each other and pray for each other so that you may be healed. The prayer of a righteous person is powerful and effective.
James 5:16

Accountability. I never liked that word. I didn't want to be accountable to anyone. I didn't want to talk to anyone about my faults. And I had a hard time admitting when I overate. I didn't want people to know that I had eaten a candy bar. Especially not if I ate two! But when I have shared my faults with someone, I found that the friend listening was understanding. The person often offered to pray with me and help me.

God tells us to be wise about who we talk to. I could go to someone with the same struggles—without really wanting to change—and that person might tell me, "It's okay." Yet that's not the answer I really needed. I once heard someone say that if a spouse is having a bad day, the other one needs to make their day better—not join the bandwagon. So I need to be careful that I'm choosing to talk to people who won't just "join the bandwagon." That I'll choose friends who will hold me accountable.

Sometimes I think I need sympathy when I really need accountability. I need someone willing to say, "What are you going to do to change that?" Someone who loves me enough to help me live a healthier life. I always told my kids as they were growing up that it's not a popularity contest; find that one friend who will be with you through thick and thin. That's all that matters.

Father, please show me which friends will hold me accountable. Bring people into my life who will be honest with me. People who want to see me healthy, who want me to be good as well as happy. In Jesus' name, amen.

by Nancy

September 28

If it is true that I have gone astray, my error remains my concern alone.
Job 19:4

The sting of death is sin, and the power of sin is the law. But thanks be to God! He gives us the victory through our Lord Jesus Christ. Therefore, my dear brothers and sisters, stand firm. Let nothing move you. Always give yourselves fully to the work of the Lord, because you know that your labor in the Lord is not in vain.
1 Corinthians 15:56–58

It seems I have a choice and a responsibility. What I choose to do with my life, with my body and mind, is my responsibility alone. I can choose the death that results from my way, or I can choose life that results from God's way. I can choose to continue in my sin, or I can turn to God, who provides a solution. I can choose to continue in my rebelliousness and willfulness, or I can surrender my will to God. It's my choice. It's my responsibility.

What God has shown me as I have struggled to overcome an eating addiction is that he wants all of me. He wants me to turn everything over to him, including my mind, my body, and my food. For a long time, I didn't realize that for most of my life I've lived for myself. But God wants me to live for him and for others. The amazing thing about finally turning my will and my life over to God is that he has in return given me so many more blessings than I could ever imagine. I've learned, ultimately, that he loves me and wants me to succeed. He wants to give me good things. And I've learned that I can't outgive God.

Father, I want to surrender it all to you. Yet I don't know if I can, so help me to do it. Whatever it takes, Lord, whatever it takes. In Jesus' name, amen.

by Debbie

September 29

You were bought at a price. Therefore, honor God with your bodies.
1 Corinthians 6:20

One of my favorite meals is a cheeseburger and fries. I could eat that a couple of times a week. Isn't it amazing how we have our favorite things and don't think twice about getting them? Even when it's not healthy. It's just so easy to just grab what I want.

I wonder what would happen if I made a healthier choice? How would I feel? I know when I make the *wrong* choice it certainly does not help my mood. It doesn't give me energy or help my day go better.

Some people talk about their love of food; I have favorites, but mainly I have bad habits that the Lord wants me to break. He wants me to walk in obedience so that I can have joy, love, and peace. When I choose something healthy to eat I feel better about myself. I also feel better physically.

My question is: Why do I eat the things I eat? Is it just a bad habit that was formed long ago? Is it really the love that I thought I had for that particular food?

It all goes back to my choices, which lead to my behavior. Sometimes I make the wrong choice, but I won't let it get me down. I'll continue on this journey toward better habits, and I'll keep working on making better choices, with God's help.

Father, I want to make better choices every day. Help me to stop and question why I'm doing the things I'm doing and help me to change them. I want to walk in obedience to you. I want to walk in health and wisdom. I want to feel good after I eat. I'm asking for your help this very moment, Lord. Thank you for helping me now. In Jesus name, amen.

by Nancy

September 30

You have set our iniquities before you, our secret sins in the light of your presence. All our days pass away under your wrath; we finish our years with a moan. Our days may come to seventy years, or eighty, if our strength endures; yet the best of them are but trouble and sorrow, for they quickly pass, and we fly away.
Psalm 90:8–10

Every once in a while, God blesses me with an epiphany, an idea so profound that it changes my life from that point forward. I think I experienced one of those this morning. In Jonathan Cahn's *Book of Mysteries*, a daily devotional, I read: ". . . there are things you'll never be able to do again, even in heaven, things you could have only done in the time you had on earth."

I already knew that intellectually. I know that life is precious. I know I shouldn't waste time, because I'm afforded so little of it. But it just hit me how many opportunities will be lost once my days on earth are over. It hit me how much time I've already wasted and how little time I have left. It makes me want to get up and redeem the time remaining to me.

I have lost so many years in overeating, in suffering the consequences of my ongoing sin. Sometimes I have longed for release from this heavy, aching body, for the thin and healthy one that will someday replace it, without realizing that I have a responsibility to eat right so that my body here and now on earth will be as healthy and able as possible so that I'll be able to do God's will now. Once I'm dead, I no longer have the opportunity to do good here on earth. I need to get moving. Now.

Father, never let me forget this lesson. Give me a sense of urgency to make things right again. To move forward. To do your will now. *Amen.*

by Debbie

Cry of Our Hearts

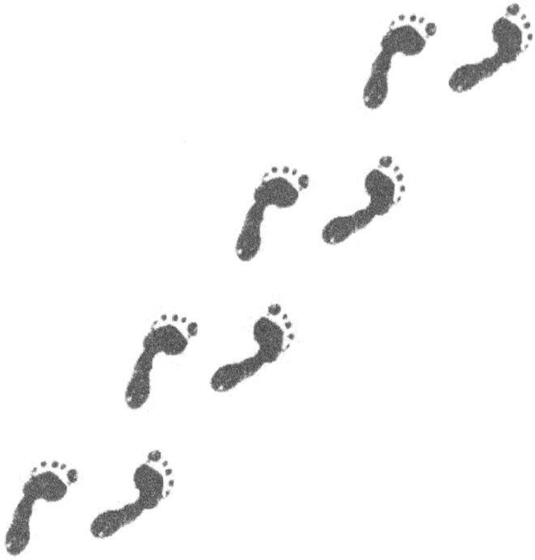

DISCIPLINE

We learn to value the practice of daily disciplines.

Cry of Our Hearts

October 1

Do not be wise in your own eyes; fear the Lord and shun evil.
This will bring health to your body and nourishment to your bones.
Proverbs 3:7–8

If you're anything like me, you can be disciplined in some areas of your life and completely out of control in others. One way that I was always disciplined was at work and at school. I was a good student. I did my homework and got good grades. At work, I always strove for excellence and often achieved it. I was always self-motivated.

And then there's food. Let's just say food wasn't my only downfall when I was younger, but I learned from most other mistakes. I became more prompt. More moral. But there's just something about food . . . I didn't realize how much of a comfort it was. I didn't realize I had become addicted, that I was eating compulsively continually. I didn't realize that at some point food had become my master.

I did realize that it was hurting my body. Making it likely I would get sick long before I got old. That if I didn't do something about my weight, I would suffer dire health consequences, and I might die far too young, at my own hand.

I finally got help by going to a twelve-step program that taught me the importance of surrendering to a Higher Power and the need to practice discipline in my eating. It was time to grow up. Learn from what I was doing wrong. Learn from others a better way of eating. I did it little by little so that I wasn't overwhelmed. That discipline with food is continually being refined. But I have to be willing, and I have to take action.

Father, help me as I learn and practice discipline over what I eat. Amen.

by Debbie

October 2

Be sober and self-controlled. Be watchful. Your adversary, the devil, walks around like a roaring lion, seeking whom he may devour.
1 Peter 5:8 WEB

Thankfully, for those of us who are born-again Christians, God tells us that one of the fruits of the Spirit is self-control. But in my experience, producing that fruit isn't automatic. In order to produce any of the fruit of the spirit in abundance ("love, joy, peace, forbearance, kindness, goodness, faithfulness, gentleness, and self-control," Galatians 5:22–23), we must stay connected to the Vine through prayer, fellowship, and study of God's word.

Jesus told his followers, "I am the vine; you are the branches. If you remain in me and I in you, you will bear much fruit; apart from me you can do nothing" (John 15:5). The Bible repeats this theme in Galatians 6:8: "Whoever sows to please their flesh, from the flesh will reap destruction; whoever sows to please the Spirit, from the Spirit will reap eternal life."

In other words, this journey toward gaining control over compulsive eating is not a one-way street. God doesn't magically arrive and deliver me from my compulsion. I must stay connected. I must sow the seeds. Only then will I reap true self-control.

For some aspects of my life, this hasn't been difficult. But with food, I have struggled repeatedly. When I do, I have to start over again fresh each morning. I'm still learning, and God is still working on increasing my self-discipline. But he is faithful when I'm faithful in turning to him before turning to the food.

Father, this has been one of the hardest things I've ever tried to do. I can't do it on my own, I know you will help me if I ask. Help me to stay connected to you and to sow the seeds of self-control every day. In Jesus' name, amen.

by Debbie

October 3

Call to me and I will answer you and tell you great and unsearchable things you do not know.
Jeremiah 33:3

I've come to realize that prayer really is the only thing that will get me through. Oh, I may try to walk the walk. I may try to say I've got it together. But if I don't spend time in communication with God, then what do I have? Just a bunch of empty air.

Losing weight is a big thing. It's not something that comes easily. It takes a lot of instruction from the Lord. A lot of patience. It's a time of losing the fat but gaining knowledge. It's a time of learning more about myself so that I'll know why I gained the weight in the first place.

But how can I learn if I don't tune into God? I could try to figure it all out on my own. So many of us are good at that. But if I do that I'll only go in circles. I won't truly know what's going on unless I let the Lord show me. And the only way He can do that is if I'm willing to spend time with him. I need to get on my knees. I need to make sure I give him time every day.

There are days when I go to God and say, "I just don't have words today, Lord." And that's fine too. I don't need to talk his leg off. I just need to sit at his feet.

Maybe he'll speak to you. Maybe he'll hold you. Maybe he'll just allow the sweet wind of peace to overtake you.

I must make that special time of day a priority. I'll put it on my calendar if I have to. But I need to spend time with my Dad today!

Abba, Father, Dad, help me make time with you a priority. Help me to make prayer a discipline in my life. In Jesus' name, amen.

by Nancy

October 4

For the Spirit God gave us does not make us timid,
but gives us power, love, and self-discipline.
2 Timothy 1:7

I know this scripture well, and I've always thought of it in terms of speaking about fear. But the last time I read it I realized it doesn't only talk about power over our anxieties. It says that God also gave us a spirit of *self-discipline.* It makes me shake my head at myself for missing it before.

Other English translations render the word self-discipline in other ways: *a sound mind*, *self-control*, and *sound judgment* are the most common. Well, I want all of that! When it comes to compulsive overeating and weight loss, I must have self-discipline to succeed.

The good news about this small bit of God's word is that it shows that God has given me a spirit that gives me self-discipline. So how do I take hold of and walk in that self-discipline? I believe it can only happen if I maintain a daily conscious contact with my Creator, the God of the Universe, who has the power to impart that spirit of self-discipline. He has the power to give me the ability to maintain self-control when I have no power of my own to do so. But I have to talk to him. I have to tell him my need. And I have to ask.

If I want guidance. If I want wisdom. If I want to stop eating compulsively and instead be disciplined in the way I eat, I must ask God to help me. I must ask. I must remember to ask.

Father, in your very word, that you sent to us as your people, you said you would give me self-discipline if I asked. So I'm asking. In Jesus' name, amen.

by Debbie

October 5

No discipline seems pleasant at the time, but painful.
Later on . . . it produces a harvest of righteousness
and peace for those who have been trained by it.
Hebrews 12:11

Consistency. It's one of the most difficult things to achieve in life. But it takes consistency to achieve any worthwhile goal, including overcoming an eating disorder or addiction or losing weight. Achieving consistency takes persistence and discipline.

Ah, yes, the "D" word: Discipline. When it came to food, I hated that word. For me, enjoying food meant a whole lot of self-indulgence and very little discipline. It wasn't until I surrendered my self-will that I was able to achieve some consistency and discipline with food. But I had to be willing to be disciplined in the way God wanted me to be disciplined. I had to be willing to do God's will when it came to food, rather than my own will.

How many times did I tell myself: "I don't think I can give that up"? Many. Once, I was discussing with a neighbor a weight-loss program I had adopted. I was talking about trying sugar-free syrup, and for some reason her response has always stayed with me. She said, "Oh, I've got to have my syrup on my pancakes." At the time, she was heavier than I was. A few years later, she died of a sudden heart attack; she was in her forties and left behind a teenage son. I wonder if she would have traded extra years for her maple syrup? I would. Or would I? I hope and pray that the result of asking God for discipline is that I get extra years to be with my loved ones.

Father, oh how foolish I have been for so very long. Thank you for showing me how insane my behavior has been with food. Let me never forget that being disciplined is worth every effort and difficulty. In Jesus' name, amen.

by Debbie

October 6

He sent out his word and healed them; he rescued them from the grave.
Psalm 107:20

And everyone who calls on the name of the Lord will be saved;
for on Mount Zion and in Jerusalem there will be deliverance,
as the Lord has said, even among the survivors whom the Lord calls.
Joel 2:32

I heard of a woman who "went to the throne room" with all her past life issues—things she had survived. After she prayed, she was delivered from that day forward. She was a new person. That was one of her life's greatest days. But she went further. She appreciated what the Lord did for her that day, yet it is only her *daily* fellowship with the Lord that keeps her in a perpetual state of deliverance.

It's not a onetime deal with God. If he delivers us, he wants it to be for life. He doesn't want us to keep grabbing it back. The way to keep it for life is to remain in fellowship with him.

Do we run to him to deliver us from our weight problems (or any problems), get excited that day, and then go back to the same ol' same ol'? Or do we ask for deliverance daily?

Many times, and to some extent still, I have asked God to help me and deliver me from this weight issue and then have gone right back to rebellious eating. Will the day come that I'll have full deliverance and no longer need to ask? It may or may not. In the meantime, it's important to ask for deliverance daily, getting into his word and fellowshipping with him consistently.

Father, help me to make fellowship with you a daily discipline. Help me to understand how important it is to my deliverance. In Jesus' name, amen.

by Nancy

October 7

Every good tree bears good fruit, but a bad tree bears bad fruit. A good tree cannot bear bad fruit, and a bad tree cannot bear good fruit. Every tree that does not bear good fruit is cut down and thrown into the fire. Thus, by their fruit you will recognize them.
Matthew 7:17–20

What can I do today to practice my faith and keep myself out of the food?

If it's Sunday, I can go to church. On any day of the week I can pray throughout the day. I can seek out some programming on TV or the Internet that will build my faith. I can do God's will by working on something I know he wants me to work on, even if it's just for a little while.

I can do my devotions, morning and night. I can exercise to keep my body in shape. I can make a call or write a letter to make amends where it might be necessary. I can listen to someone who needs my ear. I can do something for someone and make sure I do it with a good attitude. I can pray for people on my prayer list. I can send a card to a friend.

Whatever I'm working on, whether it's at my job, at home, or on a specific project, I can strive for excellence.

God wants us to be good, though he knows that we can never attain perfection. Yet goodness and self-control are fruits of the Spirit. Because God dwells in me, I can do things that I could never do on my own strength.

Father, help me to bear good fruit. I can't do it on my own power, but you have given me your Spirit, and because of that I can choose to practice my faith. Because of your love, I want to be good. Help make me a better person. Make me more and more like Jesus every day. In Jesus' name, amen.

by Debbie

October 8

When an evil spirit comes out of a man, it goes through arid places seeking rest and does not find it. Then it says, "I will return to the house I left." When it arrives, it finds the house unoccupied, swept clean and put in order. Then it goes and takes with it seven other spirits more wicked than itself, and they go in and live there. And the final condition of that man is worse than the first.
Matthew 12:43–45

The things I need to do to be obedient and eat right are not easy, because they're *work*. I'm overcoming an addiction to food, so I have to both take part in my "substance" in order to survive and still fill my needs in some way other than through the comfort of food.

The right way of meeting my needs, of course, is a closer relationship with God. But that takes time and effort too. The truth is that most people who want to lose weight don't want to make the effort. I never did! I wanted to be thin without having to give up anything or go through any pain to get there.

I think of Matthew 12:43–45. An empty house will end up worse than before, even if it's been swept clean. I have to fill up the empty house with God instead. That applies to how I deal with food. If I just go on a "diet" and give something up without replacing it with something better (God), then I'll end up worse than I was before. That's because "dieting" is temporary thinking. The changes I made to lose and keep off the weight involve discipline, because they're meant to be permanent. Self-discipline is not something that comes naturally to me. I can only achieve it by seeking God's help and power every day.

Father, teach me your ways and help me live out your discipline. Amen.

by Debbie

October 9

It teaches us to say "No" to ungodliness and worldly passions, and to live self-controlled, upright, and godly lives in this present age.
Titus 2:12

I'm really not a big eater. I don't eat a ton of food at a time. So then why do I have a hundred pounds to lose? It's because I make unwise eating choices. I eat the wrong things. I eat at the wrong times. I did a survey the other day for a weight-loss company. They focus less on the food than on behavior. I fell into almost all the categories. I eat at the wrong times. I eat out of boredom. I eat out of stress. So it's me grabbing cookies when stressed, me picking up some donuts when I'm bored.

A key to losing weight may be taking an in-depth look at my behaviors. For example, I can stop and think before I eat something. If I'm bored, I can make a conscious effort to find something else to get myself out of the boredom. If I'm stressed, a better option would be to take it to God in prayer. Eating something isn't going to take the stress away, but I know Someone who can help me with it. He's waiting for me to call out to him.

Another behavior I could work on is when I feel I need a snack, I can ask myself, "Do I really just need a glass of water?" In the past, when I drank at least sixty ounces of water a day, I didn't eat nearly as many snacks. I just wasn't hungry. What I don't have to ask myself is whether God can help me, because I know he can. And will—if I remember to ask.

Father, please help me change my behavior. Open my eyes to see what changes I need to make. Help me rely on you, and not on the food. Forgive me, Father. In Jesus' name, amen.

by Nancy

October 10

Whatever you do, do your work heartily, as for the Lord and not for people, knowing that it is from the Lord that you will receive the reward of the inheritance. It is the Lord Christ whom you serve.
Colossians 3:23–24

In my weak human nature, I always want to find an easier, softer way. Trouble is, it doesn't exist. Almost everything worth having takes work to achieve, and that includes recovery from any addiction. To quote Westley in the movie *The Princess Bride*, "Anyone who says differently is selling something."

The good news is that it may not take as much work as you might think. One reason for that is that part of this journey has been developing a dependence on God, because in the weakness of my human nature, he demonstrates his strength.

Yet I do things differently now than I did in the past. I take specific actions every day that are becoming a part of a recovery discipline designed to keep me from ever going back to the misery I felt when I was at my top weight.

It's worth it to spend a few extra minutes of my time every day to ensure that I stay in recovery. It's worth it to weigh and measure my food. It's worth it to eat meals according to a regular schedule most of the time. It's worth it to read labels. It's worth it to have a devotional time in the mornings and evenings. It's worth it to pray before I eat and ask God to make it enough. It's worth it, because the rewards are greater than the sacrifice.

Father, help me to continue to be diligent in recovery. Let me never forget what it used to be like so that I'll do whatever it takes to never go back to where I was. Never let me forget that it takes disciplined action to recover from addiction. In Jesus' name, amen.

by Debbie

October 11

Have nothing to do with godless myths and old wives' tales; rather, train yourself to be godly. For physical training is of some value, but godliness has value for all things, holding promise for both the present life and the life to come.
1 Timothy 4:7–8

God has been working on me a lot in the past couple of years. He has asked quite a bit of me. I liken it to the physical training the Apostle Paul is talking about in this scripture, but the Lord is instead training me spiritually. Though it doesn't come naturally to me, he's been teaching me spiritual disciplines in the way athletes learn physical discipline.

I've learned some physical discipline too. I've changed my diet significantly, eliminating almost all refined sugar and most white flour as well. I do about ten minutes of core-strengthening exercises almost every morning that I hope are of some benefit.

Yet without the spiritual disciplines I've learned, these new physical disciplines would never have occurred. Every day I read twelve-step literature. I also read a biblical devotional and study scripture. I didn't do that before starting back on my weight-loss journey, but without doing those things, I never would have found the strength to begin or continue with the physical changes. And God isn't finished with me yet. There's more training to come. He's nudging me toward a more disciplined prayer life. And it's all linked to overcoming compulsive eating.

What am I training for? Whatever he asks of me. And it's all designed to make me more like him.

Father, make me willing to listen to and obey your instruction. Help me to be disciplined in the ways you are leading me. In Jesus' name, amen.

by Debbie

October 12

Blessed is the man who remains steadfast under trial,
for when he has stood the test he will receive the crown of life,
which God has promised to those who love him.
James 1:12 ESV

Do you not know that in a race all the runners run, but only one gets the prize? Run in such a way as to get the prize. Everyone who competes in the games goes into strict training. They do it to get a crown that will not last, but we do it to get a crown that will last forever.
1 Corinthians 9:24–25

Sometimes I feel I just can't try anymore. I just can't do it. With everything within me, I want to give up. Then something comes along to show me why I need to keep going. My grandkids are a huge motivator for me.

We all have those things that we need to keep fighting for. Those things that will cause us to stay in the fight.

This is not an easy thing. Overcoming the compulsion to overeat will try us on every level. We will have ups and downs.

But I know that I will continue to press onward. I will remain steadfast so that I can be here for my grandkids.

What is that one thing in your life? Maybe you have more than one. Let's press on and remain steadfast, and we'll receive the prize.

Father, I pray that I can keep pressing onward. I pray that I'll remain steadfast and earn the prize. The prize of better health. The prize of living longer so I can be with my family longer. The prize of knowing that I ran the race for you, and I did it! Thank you, Lord, for never giving up on me. Thank you for always being here for me. In Jesus' name, amen.

by Nancy

October 13

I gave them this command:
Obey me, and I will be your God and you will be my people.
Walk in obedience to all I command you, that it may go well with you.
Jeremiah 7:23

No matter how long I have been on this journey toward a healthy body weight, the false hunger sometimes returns. And sometimes when I've finished the food on my plate, it feels like it's not enough. There is something broken about my body in that there is often a delay between the time I finish eating and the time I feel full.

What happened in the past is that if I kept eating because my brain and body were telling me I wasn't yet satisfied, a little while later I actually felt uncomfortably full. Overly full. One of the things I have had to do to overcome this disconnect with not feeling full when I should is to measure my food and stop when I've finished eating the serving that I know should satisfy me.

Then I often have to pray, "Lord, please let this food be enough for me right now." Then I wait until I feel full, which typically only takes a few minutes. It works, because when I take the right action (which for me is stopping even before I *feel* full), God honors my prayers.

Obedience isn't easy, and most of the time it's not very fun. Sometimes I don't even understand why I need to obey, I just know I need to do it.

Father, you have shown me what kinds of food I need to stay away from, how much I should eat, and how often. Now that I know what you want me to do, help me to obey. Give me the strength to eat the way you want me to eat. Help me to be disciplined the way you want me to be. In Jesus' name, amen.

by Debbie

October 14

Though the righteous fall seven times, they rise again.
Proverbs 24:16

But those who hope in the Lord will renew their strength.
They will soar on wings like eagles; they will run
and not grow weary, they will walk and not be faint.
Isaiah 40:31

Learning how to eat healthy and be satisfied with reduced portions has been a challenge, though that is a lot of what it has taken to lose weight. In fact, sometimes it's been a rollercoaster ride. Sometimes I succeed and I'm down. Then I eat too much one evening, and that puts me on an upward trend.

In the past, before I turned this weight-loss journey over to God, in the face of one failure I would give up and go back to *all* my old habits. The difference this time around is that I have persisted. If I fall off the horse, I get right back in the saddle. God helps me to recognize what I've done and tells me to try again. And I do. If my clothes get a little tighter and I step on the scale to see whether it's just my imagination (usually it's not), if the scale says I'm up a few pounds it means I need to return to being diligent about what I eat. And I do.

Maybe I fell down because I was careless. Maybe I was willful and have eaten something the Lord has told me is not good for me. Sometimes I need to examine why I did what I did. And sometimes I just need to forget about what happened, get back up, and go back to doing the things that work.

Father, never let me forget that you want me to keep doing the right thing even when I fall. Then help me to get back up and do it. In Jesus' name, amen.

by Debbie

October 15

Do you not know that you are a temple of God and that the Spirit of God dwells in you? If anyone destroys the temple of God, God will destroy that person; for the temple of God is holy, and that is what you are.
1 Corinthians 3:16–17

God is rooting for me. He is rooting for all of us. I can see him up there with his pom poms, cheering with the angels. He wants us healthy. He wants us strong and able to further his kingdom. He just plain wants us happy in our own skin. So why not go to the one who is our biggest fan? Our biggest supporter?

I really need to follow through with my plan that I was going to spend time each morning going to the Lord and praying specifically for this. And in the afternoon if I feel that I'm going to get out of control with my eating, I'll go to him once again.

My brother-in-law quit smoking in the same way. Every time the temptation came, he went to his room or a quiet spot and got with God. I can do the same thing.

I also quit smoking. At that time I did it by finding every scripture that the Lord showed me that talked about what he thinks of sin and applying it to my smoking habit. It's time to dig out the scriptures he has already shown me about the sin of overeating.

Choosing to seek God when I'm tempted is something I can learn and practice. It can become a discipline in my life.

Father, help me to see sin as sin, no matter what it is. And then help me to become disciplined enough to seek you first instead of the pleasure of the sin. In Jesus' name, amen.

by Nancy

October 16

*In the morning, Lord, you hear my voice; in the morning
I lay my requests before you and wait expectantly.*
Psalm 5:3

Let the morning bring me word of your unfailing love, for I have put my trust in you. Show me the way I should go, for to you I entrust my life. Rescue me from my enemies, Lord, for I hide myself in you. Teach me to do your will, for you are my God; may your good Spirit lead me on level ground.
Psalm 143:8–10

*I remember the days of long ago; I meditate on
all your works and consider what your hands have done.*
Psalm 143:5

It's just as important to start my day listening to God (meditating) as it is to pray (ask him for something). I once heard someone share that she spends two minutes in that kind of meditation every day and that, inevitably, makes the difference between a bad day and a good one.

My biggest problem in that regard is my "ADD" mind; my thoughts wander of their own accord and never seem to stop, so it's always a challenge. But I'm willing to try, over and over again.

It does help to have things quiet and to start with reading some kind of devotional that includes a scripture reading. It's never a waste of time to start my day meditating on God's word and praying for wisdom and guidance for the day.

Father, help me to not only remember to ask you for what I need, but also to listen for the answers you have for me. Help me learn to be disciplined in prayer. In Jesus' name, amen.

by Debbie

October 17

Let the wise listen and add to their learning,
and let the discerning get guidance.
Proverbs 1:5

There's a saying Americans have: You have to pay your dues. To me it means that I might have to start off in a place that's uncomfortable so that I can learn. Then I move up to the next step, and I learn some more. Each job, each duty, each thing I learn is a little better than the one before. Maybe the result is that it's a little less uncomfortable. A little less difficult. A little easier.

That's because I've paid my dues. I've learned the lessons. I've gained the experience I needed to move up to the next step.

I have found this to be true with my weight-loss journey. When I first started I was skeptical that it could even work. I'd been failing at diets for so long, I had basically given up. But then I saw people who had lost weight and kept it off for years. Even decades. And I realized that if they could do it, maybe I could too. Especially after hearing their stories—since most of them had started off just as hopeless as I was.

Little by little I listened. I learned. I took action. And I began to change. And I'm still changing. Still learning. Still listening.

I can look at life as if it's a rollercoaster ride, where I'm just looking for thrills. Or I can look at life like a school, where I'm meant to learn from everything I go through. God has given me a journey, and learning how to respond to food in a sane manner (as opposed to total insanity) is one of those lessons God wants me to learn. So I have to pay my dues and learn, little by little.

Father, help me to be content where I am, learning what you want to teach me. Help me to be a good student and patiently pay my dues. Amen.

by Debbie

October 18

When you sit down to eat with a ruler, observe carefully what is before you, and put a knife to your throat if you are given to appetite. Do not desire his delicacies, for they are deceptive food.
Proverbs 23:1–3

Every athlete exercises self-control in all things. They do it to receive a perishable wreath, but we an imperishable. So I do not run aimlessly; I do not box as one beating the air. But I discipline my body and keep it under control, lest after preaching to others I myself should be disqualified.
I Corinthians 9:25–27 ESV

Is something taking God's place in my life? When I think of that question, I feel broken inside. All I can do is fall to my knees and say, "I'm sorry, Lord!" I know that I have put food where he should be. Can we see when we've done that?

Food is such a basic part of life that we often just cannot fathom that we could possibly put it before God. After all, we need it for nourishment. We need it to live. But do we need it for satisfaction? Do we need it for fun? Do we need it for friendship?

Life is more than food. There's so much life out there. God wants us to live it to the fullest. He wants us to be joyful and healthy. And the two together—joy and health—make for a pretty good life.

Can you feel it in the pit of your stomach? Can you feel the brokenness? The desire to repent and cry out, "ABBA FATHER, please forgive me"?

Father, forgive me for all the junk I have eaten today and in the past. Make me willing, and then teach me to be disciplined. Lord, guide me to eat to live and not to live to eat. In Jesus' name, amen!

by Nancy

October 19

For everything in the world—the lust of the flesh, the lust of the eyes, and the pride of life—comes not from the Father but from the world.
1 John 2:16

Bringing into captivity every thought to the obedience of Christ.
2 Corinthians 10:5 KJV

I sometimes get feelings of envy when I see TV commercials about food. Or at other times when I see people eating normal things, like mashed potatoes and gravy (my personal kryptonite), either in person or in a TV show or movie. I had to go through a period of mourning over "losing" certain foods. Eliminating sugar and (for me) most white flour all at once is a big change. Plus, the number and kinds of foods on my list of the "trigger" foods I have been willing to give up has grown over the years.

But I knew I needed to eliminate sugar or else I would continue to consume too much food at each meal, and between meals, and I didn't want to do that anymore. I attribute that to an allergy to sugar—much the same as an alcoholic is allergic to the ethanol in spirits. Giving up refined sugar has worked, because I can usually tell when I'm full now, and most of the time I'm satisfied when I'm done eating.

When I do get those feelings of envy now, I deal with them by dismissing the thought with another: "It's just not worth it." In that way, the feelings are fleeting—they leave me quickly. And I attribute that to God's grace creating discipline in my life and in my thoughts.

Father, give me strength to continue rejecting thoughts that don't come from you. Help me to discipline my thoughts. In Jesus' name, amen.

by Debbie

October 20

Yes, I will bless the Lord and not forget the glorious things he does for me. He forgives all my sins. He heals me. He ransoms me from hell. He surrounds me with loving-kindness and tender mercies.
Psalm 103:2–4

Do not conform to the pattern of this world, but be transformed by the renewing of your mind. Then you will be able to test and approve what God's will is—his good, pleasing, and perfect will.
Romans 12:2

I came to a point in this journey toward recovery from food addiction that I had to ask God to remove those defects of character that keep me from living according to his purpose for me. One of my greatest shortcomings is fear, so I asked God to replace that with a confidence and boldness that I would never naturally have on my own.

I also discovered that it is the defects of self-will, ego, and denial that always lead me back into self-destruction with food. So I must also pray to be free of those.

This is not something that will happen overnight. And it won't happen unless I take consistent, self-disciplined actions. Not just once in a while, but repeatedly, every day. In order to recover, I must repeat, every day, the things that worked the day before. I must also learn from the things that didn't work so that I can let go of them.

Father, make me willing to give up those things that you want me to give up—for your glory and for my own benefit and for the benefit of those whose lives I touch. In Jesus' name, amen.

by Debbie

October 21

They promise freedom to everyone. But they are merely slaves of filthy living, because people are slaves of whatever controls them.
2 Peter 2:19 CEV

I've heard that it takes twenty-one days to form a new habit. I'm unsure how long it really takes, but I do know that for each day that I make a better choice and keep repeating it—eventually my brain will tell me that it's normal. I really am the slave to what controls me. It's up to me to break that control, with God's help. It helps to learn one thing at a time.

I started with telling myself that I won't keep candy in the house. In the past I made a deal with myself that I wouldn't have any candy in the house, but I would allow myself a candy bar while I was out shopping. What I noticed after a while is that I "forgot" to buy a candy bar. It just wasn't normal anymore for me to grab one. In that way, I can form good habits.

I also once had a conversation with myself. I wanted a snack, but I told myself to wait ten minutes. Then if I wanted a snack, I could have one. Half an hour later, I remembered the snack. So I repeated what I'd done earlier; I told myself if I still wanted a snack in ten minutes, I could have one. In that way, I had one snack that night compared to the three I normally had.

Little habits often become big habits. And breaking little habits can help to break big ones. Today, I can be obedient to God in choosing to break a little habit.

Father, show me what you want me to change and what you want me to do to break a bad habit or create a good habit. Lord, whatever it is, guide me. Help me find the new normal. Help me create the habits I'll need to walk the road of victory. In Jesus' name, amen.

by Nancy

October 22

Do not be anxious about anything, but in everything by prayer and supplication with thanksgiving let your requests be made known to God.
Philippians 4:6

Likewise the Spirit helps us in our weakness. For we do not know what to pray for as we ought, but the Spirit himself intercedes for us with groanings too deep for words.
Romans 8:26

One of the things I'm really bad at is long prayers. I'm pretty good for a few minutes, but if I tried to practice the kind of praying that Daniel did or Jesus did, I fear I would fail utterly. I seem to have some kind of "prayer ADD." I have difficulty keeping my mind focused for more than a few minutes at a time.

So what can I do to get better about that? Like anything, it will take practice. In the meantime, I can ask God to bring my thoughts to him more often. I can concentrate on how much I need him to help me throughout my day. I can talk to God, even if it's briefly, throughout each day. I can remember that God wants to be my friend.

I can pray that God will help me to eat cleanly and according to his will. I can pray that what I eat will be enough today and that I won't feel compelled to go back for more. The important thing is that I pray. And pray again. And pray some more. That I practice praying, every day, many times a day.

Father, put into my mind and heart the need to pray without ceasing. Don't let me forget how important it is to make that connection with you every day. Help me to make a practice of prayer so that I can continue to do your will. In Jesus' name, amen.

by Debbie

October 23

He predestined us for adoption to sonship through Jesus Christ,
in accordance with his pleasure and will.
Ephesians 1:5

But when the set time had fully come, God sent his Son, born of a woman, born under the law, to redeem those under the law, that we might receive adoption to sonship. Because you are his sons, God sent the Spirit of his Son into our hearts, the Spirit who calls out, "Abba, Father." So you are no longer a slave, but God's child; and since you are his child, God has made you also an heir.
Galatians 4:4–7

Do you not know that your bodies are temples of the Holy Spirit, who is in you, whom you have received from God? You are not your own.
1 Corinthians 6:19

Being in God's family is such a blessing. It really is a wonderful reminder that God cares for each of us and that I am somehow also part of his plan. That as a member of his family, he will care for me like a daughter and that his planned inheritance for me is manifold riches in eternity, in all senses of the word. If he cares so much for me, then he also must care about the health and well-being of my body as well as my spirit. If that's true, then how can I care anything less than he does? If I'm not disciplined about the food I put in my body, then what exactly am I saying to God about this wonderful body he gave me to live out my life in?

Father, help me to think of my body as a precious gift, and give me the strength to treat it with value and respect. In Jesus' name, amen.

by Debbie

October 24

Each of you should give what you have decided in your heart to give, not reluctantly or under compulsion, for God loves a cheerful giver.
2 Corinthians 9:7

Sometimes I have to check myself and see if I'm wanting more from God than what I'm willing to give. I can't outgive God, but I can ask myself what I can offer him. I can offer him my time. I can offer him my tithes. I can offer him my obedience.

Obedience is a hard word to swallow. When I think of obedience, I think of when I was a kid having to obey my parents. If I didn't do what they wanted, it was not a pretty sight. I tend to want to link that with God. But if I can change my mindset, I'll recognize that all God wants is to keep me safe. He wants to keep me healthy. He only wants good for me. So then is the word obedience really that bad? Was it bad back when I was a kid?

The truth is that God is willing to let us have our own way. We have free will, and that's where I have to ask myself: Am I harming myself with my choices? Is it worth going against what God has instructed me—us—to do in order to have the happiest, safest, and healthiest life possible within his will for me?

There's so much joy to be experienced when I do the right thing. When I make the right choices, I feel true happiness. When I choose wrong, I don't feel so good—mentally or physically.

Father, I pray that today will be a day of recognizing what I can do for you. Jesus, I want to give my all to you. All my thoughts. All my actions. All my choices. All my food. Thank you, Lord, for loving me. Thank you, Lord, for wanting the best for me. In Jesus' name, amen.

by Nancy

October 25

My grace is sufficient for you, for my power is made perfect in weakness.
2 Corinthians 12:9

Isn't it ironic that the problem that I find most besetting, most troublesome, and the hardest to overcome is the very same one that has caused the most emotional and spiritual growth in my life? For me, that problem is compulsive overeating. By working toward recovering from the addiction of compulsive eating, I have discovered much worth learning.

I have learned obedience to God, trust in God, and dependence on God. I have learned that God's strength is made perfect in my weakness, that I must be in contact with God daily about this overwhelming problem.

I have also learned that I can rejoice in my current circumstances no matter what they are. I have learned about the power of forgiveness—God's forgiveness of me, my need to ask for forgiveness from others, and the need to forgive those who have harmed me. I have learned the importance of doing more than just asking for God's help, but the need to act in obedience first. I have learned that discipline is not a dirty word. And so much more.

Should I be praising and thanking God for this weakness? Why not? Working so hard to overcome it has made me a better (though far from perfect) person. And as I let him, God continues to make me a better person every day.

Father, I never thought I could thank you for making it so easy for my body to retain extra weight. Nor did I think I could ever thank you for this thorn in the flesh that makes me think food is the comfort for every problem. But I can thank you now, because this problem has made me turn to you as my God, my strength, my help, and my comfort. Thank you. In Jesus' name, amen.

by Debbie

October 26

Nevertheless, the righteous will hold to their ways,
and those with clean hands will grow stronger.
Job 17:9

When I was in grad school, one of the things we were asked to do is take the online Strengths Survey from the VIA Institute on Character. (You can take it too; it's free.) This instrument measures twenty-four dimensions of character, ranking strengths based on answers to a set of questions. I was interested to learn that number four on my list is *perseverance.* (Perhaps not surprising is that the last on my list is self-regulation, a.k.a., self-discipline.)

If perseverance is one of my main strengths, then why in the past haven't I been able to "stick to a diet"? I think in part it's because I respond differently to food than other people. There are some foods I'm allergic to. Ironically, those are the very foods I crave the most, the ones I find most addictive.

Another aspect of my struggle is that—because food is one of my greatest weaknesses—I can't rely on my own strength to overcome my compulsiveness with it. I must rely on a power greater than my own, God.

Once I recognized those weaknesses and changed the way I relate to food—then I could leverage the strength of perseverance. I can persevere in reaching out to God for strength and wisdom. I can persevere in choosing not to partake of those foods that are my downfall. I can reject my lack of self-discipline and ask God to help me. I don't have to continue on without hope, because now God has become my hope and strength.

Father, please give me the strength to persevere in self-discipline with my food and in a discipline of daily reaching out to you for help. Amen.

by Debbie

October 27

When an impure spirit comes out of a person, it goes through arid places seeking rest and does not find it. Then it says, "I will return to the house I left." When it arrives, it finds the house swept clean and put in order. Then it goes and takes seven other spirits more wicked than itself, and they go in and live there. And the final condition of that person is worse than the first.
Luke 11:24–26

I think of this scripture often when I think about overcoming addiction of any kind, though mine happens to be to sugar and a few other trigger foods. How many times have I prayed and asked God to give me the motivation to lose weight? Many. I started on weight-loss journeys many times in my life. As a teen I tried Atkins. As an adult I've tried Weight Watchers, TOPS, Jenny Craig, Nutrisystem, and Kaiser's Freedom from Fat. And many times I tried to just do it on my own. Some of them worked for a time, but never more than a few weeks.

As my addiction progressed, it got harder and harder to stick to anything. At one point I couldn't even make it through one day of eating sensibly. The demons always returned, often with a vengeance. What has made the difference this time? First, I treated my addiction like the three-legged stool that it is: physical, emotional, and spiritual. And I *treated* it. I replaced the emptiness with action. I followed a plan that deals with my entire being. So my house is no longer just swept clean. It's full of planning and discipline, daily reading and study, fellowship, prayer, and dependency on God for the strength I don't have myself.

Father, you have filled in the empty places in my soul with your loving presence, with your Holy Spirit. It's such a gift! Thank you! Amen.

by Debbie

October 28

Because of the Lord's great love we are not consumed, for his compassions never fail. They are new every morning; great is your faithfulness.
Lamentations 3:22–23

I got some news that I never wanted to hear from my doctor: "You have diabetes." I know that many people have managed their diabetes for years, but I experienced it as *another* diagnosis. I just get tired of getting one diagnosis after another. I long to live a healthy life. To hear good news from the doctor.

I talked to my mom, who has diabetes. She was of great help and encouragement. I ultimately decided to manage it myself. (I don't recommend that for everyone. My numbers were low enough that taking that action seemed appropriate. Please follow your doctor's advice.)

I told my mom, "I guess I've had my last hoorah." She told me, "No, you have to think of it as a new beginning." Then someone else told me, "It's a new day."

When I hear negative news, I have a choice about how to react. Will I choose a woe-is-me attitude? Or take it as a new beginning? With things to learn. As the start of a healthier lifestyle.

God tells us not to look back. His mercies are new every morning. It's just one more example of how great God is. He has promised us new mornings. I just need to latch onto him and walk in that newness. Oh, how my Father wants to help me with the new walk I'm taking. He longs to help me defeat diabetes.

Am I so set in my ways that I can't walk in the new? Sometimes new is good. Sometimes change is good.

Father, you want to put new things in my life. Guide me into newer, healthier ways. Into a more joyful way of living. In Jesus' name, amen.

by Nancy

October 29

"Is not this the kind of fasting I have chosen . . . Is it not to share your food with the hungry and to provide the poor wanderer with shelter—when you see the naked, to clothe them, and not to turn away from your own flesh and blood? Then your light will break forth like the dawn, and your healing will quickly appear; then your righteousness will go before you, and the glory of the Lord will be your rear guard. Then you will call, and the Lord will answer; you will cry for help, and he will say: Here am I.
Isaiah 58:6–9

All my adult life in church I've heard about the importance of fasting on occasion. Trouble is, I never understood its purpose. The one time I did fast at length, I didn't experience a benefit. And as a compulsive overeater, I had trouble even thinking about trying again. After that, the only time I fasted, though even then I did it begrudgingly, was for medical purposes.

Plus, though I don't qualify, for anyone who has experienced anorexia or bulimia, fasting can be dangerous. Sometimes even compulsive eating (which is a problem for me), can sometimes translate into restricting food instead, so for those of us with issues with food, fasting must be done thoughtfully and carefully.

Yet this passage from Isaiah showed me another way. We fast from food at times to humble ourselves, to focus our attention on God and spend time with him, to focus on prayer, and to show God that we're sincere about something we're asking for. But we can also do it to benefit others. We can give up something and give it to those who need it instead. And in this scripture, we are promised a breakthrough and blessings when we do.

Father, if this is a discipline you want me to take part in, please show me. Show me when you want me to fast and for which purposes. Amen.

by Debbie

October 30

And if your eye causes you to stumble, gouge it out and throw it away. It is better for you to enter life with one eye than to have two eyes and be thrown into the fire of hell.
Matthew 18:9

Christians today don't often quote that scripture from Matthew, because it's stark, harsh, and scary. Yet there are several important spiritual principles in it. First, those are red-letter words. Jesus said them. That means I should pay extra attention. In other words, I shouldn't take sin lightly; it's serious business with serious consequences, and that includes my sin of willful overeating. Second, I should do whatever it takes to keep from sinning, including removing from my life anything that will continually put me in the way of something that tempts me.

I learned a new slogan today that's similar to Jesus' words: "If you don't want to slip, stay away from slippery places." When it comes to overeating, there are a lot of slippery places—for me those "places" are typically certain kinds of food. I now know that I need to completely abstain from refined sugar (that includes all forms of sugar, including corn syrup). There are other foods that tend to trip me up as well. Most white flour. Fried and mashed potatoes. A lot of traditional "comfort" foods. If I don't want to slip, I need to stay away from my "slippery" foods. Completely. It's a matter of knowing the importance of keeping myself from sin. And when I can't do it in my own power, instead of trying to lean on the willpower I don't have, I need to lean on God's power. It's only in relying on God that I can succeed.

Father, remind me how awful sin really is, including the sin of gluttony, and keep me from it at all times. In Jesus' name, amen.

by Debbie

October 31

Then, because so many people were coming and going that they did not even have a chance to eat, he said to them, "Come with me by yourselves to a quiet place and get some rest."
Mark 6:31

For he knows our frame; he remembers that we are dust.
Psalm 103:14 ESV

He restores my soul.
Psalm 23:3

There's an acronym used in twelve-step programs: HALT, which stands for Hungry, Angry, Lonely, Tired. If I'm any of those things, I'm more likely, when I'm tempted, to give in to eating too much or to eating things that aren't good for me.

This is most likely to happen when I'm tired or feeling even a little under the weather. When I'm weary is the time I want the most comfort, and food has been my comfort for so long that's the time when it's hardest for me to say no to myself.

What it means is that I need to take care of myself. I need to make sure I don't get to the point of being ravenously hungry. I need to do something about being angry before it festers and causes me to turn to food for comfort. I need to reach out to a friend if I'm lonely. And I need to rest if I'm tired. I also need to watch that I don't let myself get burned out.

God wants us to take care of ourselves, and he's willing and able to help us do that. It's okay to allow time to meet my own needs. In fact, in order to succeed at eating right, it's imperative.

Father, when I work too hard, remind me to rest. When I'm close to being burned out, let me know before it goes too far. Restore my soul. Amen.

by Debbie

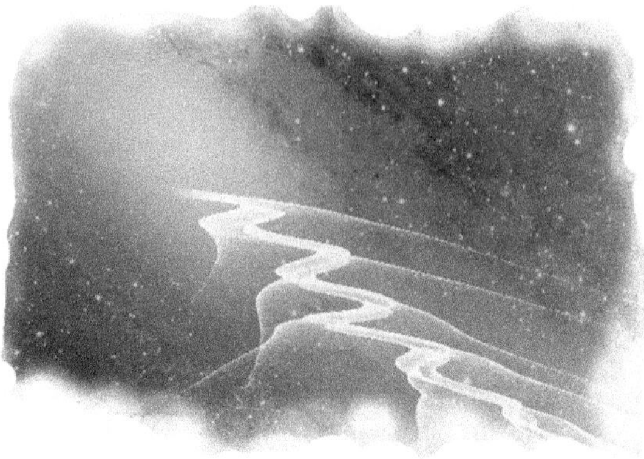

AWARENESS

We learn to spend intentional daily time with God.

Cry of Our Hearts

November 1

On his robe and on his thigh he has this name written:
King of Kings and Lord of Lords.
Revelation 19:16

I've been feeling more and more that I just want to go to the King. I want to lay it all down before him. I want to lay down at his feet. I feel like I don't have a lot to bring, but he feels like I have a lot to offer. He sees me as special, and he wants me to just be with him. He wants to sit and chat. He wants to comfort me. He wants to support me in everything.

I need so much support with this weight-loss journey, and he is the One who can help me through every mistake I make. He won't judge me for them. He loves me, even with my screw-ups. He'll guide me back to the right path and love me through it. He won't have harsh words for me. He won't yell at me. He'll gently, in a still, small voice, guide me back to where I need to be.

What would I be without him? I get so weary of the fight, but he doesn't. He picks me up and carries me through the toughest times. He guides me, showing me what to do next.

I really don't have much to bring him, but he has the world to bring to me. If only I'll let him. If only I'll go to him with everything.

Father, please remind me to be in constant communication with you through the day. Help me to speak to you as if you're right next to me. Help me to be completely raw and open with you. Help me not try to hide things. To not be so discouraged that I think you no longer care for me. Help me know that you're right here with me. You're listening to every word I say. Even when I'm angry, help me know that I can share that anger with you. Thank you, Lord. I love you more than I could ever have imagined. In Jesus' name, amen.

by Nancy

November 2

The kingdom of heaven is like treasure hidden in a field.
When a man found it, he hid it again, and then in his joy
went and sold all he had and bought that field.
Matthew 13:44

What makes me eat? Do I eat to live or live to eat? Do I eat when under stress? Why? I've been thinking about why I choose to eat when I'm under stress (or feeling any other emotion). I mean, what is it about food that comforts me?

Sometimes I think we can look into our past and find the answer. One thing I remember doing when I was younger was going out to eat with my mom. It was a rare occasion, as things were tight financially then. Those precious times were special to me.

It makes me wonder if that's why I run to food when I'm upset or hurting. When money is tight, do I feel I have to eat now before there's nothing left? Is food how I make my memories?

There has to be a reason why I have chosen food. Some people exercise. Some people do drugs. Some people drink alcohol. Some people sleep. Some people fight. There has to be a reason why I choose food. Yet it isn't enough just to see what it is. I have to find a way to replace it. I need to make God my treasure instead of the food. He needs to become what's precious to me so that I turn to him instead.

Father, please help me to see that choosing food is the wrong way. Please put that knowledge deep down in my soul so that I'll never forget it. So that it will become second nature to me. Help me to see that to choose you is the better way. Help me to see you like the man saw the treasure in the field, so that when I see how wonderful you really are that I'll choose you instead of the food every time. In Jesus' name, amen.

by Nancy

November 3

But blessed is the one who trusts in the Lord, whose confidence is in him. They will be like a tree planted by the water that sends out its roots by the stream.
Jeremiah 17:7–8

For I am the Lord your God who takes hold of your right hand and says to you, Do not fear; I will help you.
Isaiah 41:13

My thoughts around food are sometimes still a little off—a little insane. I sometimes still crave food when I'm not truly hungry. Food has been "the answer" to my problems for so long that it's almost an automatic response to turn to it instead of to what I really need. And what does that mean? It means I'm craving something else and still looking to food to meet that inner need, that inner emptiness.

It also means making a conscious effort to do something different from what I've always done before.

What is the answer, then? I can pray more. In my daily routine I can become more aware of God's glory and power. I can ask God to show me the truth and to help me be honest with myself. I can ask for God's direction. I can spend a little time each day worshipping God and communing with him in the Spirit. I can ask God to be enough for me.

Father, please help relieve me of this obsession I still sometimes feel—it would be to your glory if you can help me overcome it and turn to you. If I can achieve the weight loss I desire with your help, then I can give you the glory for giving me the power to do something that I could never do on my own. In Jesus' name, amen.

by Debbie

November 4

Search me, God, and know my heart; test me and know my anxious thoughts. See if there is any offensive way in me, and lead me in the way everlasting.
Psalm 139:23–24

I believe that this weight-loss journey is not just about eating less. There are reasons why I overeat. Consciously or subconsciously, I'm hurting myself. I've heard it said that overeating is a slow suicide. So why am I doing it? Is it because I come from an abused past? Because I'm in a hurtful situation? Do I see myself as unworthy of any good in my life? Am I hiding under the fat? Do I want to avoid negative feelings?

Whatever the reasons, God wants to work through each of them. As I have gone through this journey, there have been many issues in my life that God has had to bring out and deal with.

I have had to work through the abuses in my past. To work through issues in my personal life. To work with deep-down, hidden anger. To work through many fears. To work through wrong attitudes. I have had to forgive even when I didn't want to, including forgiving myself. I even had to give up a lot of my "mannerisms" that have tried to make me become who I am not.

I had to realize that I don't need to impress anyone but the Father. I have to stretch my wings and attempt to fly. Sometimes I have fallen, but the Father has always been there to swoop under me with wings like an eagle—and catch me. So I have to be willing to be a work in progress. That is how I get through!

Father, help me better understand my reasons for eating. Even more important, lead me on a path that will allow me to stop hurting myself. In Jesus' name, amen.

by Nancy

November 5

We demolish arguments and every pretension that sets itself up against the knowledge of God, and we take captive every thought to make it obedient to Christ.
2 Corinthians 10:5

What do I think of myself? And how important is that to my weight loss? I consider myself a shy person. I'm the one in the back row at church or events. I try to sneak in quietly so that I don't draw attention to myself. Witnessing? That scares me. I get to know someone before I ever mention God.

It goes back to self-perception. How do I see myself? Is that what God wants me to see? God made some of us to be introverts for a purpose, just as he made outgoing people who aren't afraid of anything. Our self-perceptions affect the way we handle ourselves, handle situations, and carry ourselves. They affect our lifestyle and our relationships.

I, for one, have a hard time being around people who complain a lot. I'm not talking about going through a difficult season when it helps to talk it through. But I've known people who never change. They're always negative about life and everything around them. But I also need to have compassion, because I believe chronic complainers don't see themselves too highly. They have some inner work they need to do. Like most of us. Like me.

Father, help me not to play a negative mind game. Help me see myself in a clearer light, in the light of Jesus. Each time I want to put myself down or see myself differently from the way you do, help me to take that thought into captivity. Help me to see the potential you see in me. Help me to have a healthy image of myself, as the one you created. In Jesus' name, amen.

by Nancy

November 6

Now when [Elisha's] attendant had risen early and gone out, behold, an army with horses and chariots was circling the city. And his servant said to him, "This is hopeless, my master! What are we to do?" And he said, "Do not be afraid, for those who are with us are greater than those who are with them." Then Elisha prayed and said, "Lord, please, open his eyes so that he may see." And the Lord opened the servant's eyes, and he saw; and behold, the mountain was full of horses and chariots of fire."
2 Kings 6: 15–17

I was waiting to see the doctor for a routine visit. I looked around the exam room to pass the time and thought, "Now I know what they mean by clinical." There were no decorations on the wall—no pictures, nothing to entertain an impatiently waiting patient. I looked up at the ceiling, because sometimes doctors will put pictures up there for their patients to see while they're lying back on the examination table. Nope, nothing there, either.

The physician's assistant came in, asked some questions and took my blood pressure. After she left, I looked around some more. I glanced up and was astonished to realize that there were two shiny, colorful mobiles hanging from the ceiling. I had looked directly at the same place earlier. Why hadn't I noticed them before? I knew immediately this was a lesson, and I prayed, "Lord, what is it you want me to learn here?" The answer was simple: *It's easy to be blind about a lot of things. When you're looking for something else, you won't always see what's really there. Let me open your eyes to the truth, and you will finally see it.*

Father, open my eyes to what you would have me see. Let me not be blinded by my own opinions and assumptions. Let me see, Lord, always, what is truly there. Let your truth reign in my heart and mind. In Jesus' name, amen.

by Debbie

November 7

What benefit did you reap at that time from the things you are now ashamed of? Those things result in death!
Romans 6:21

In the Christian romance novel *Beyond the Shadows*, the heroine's husband talks a lot about overcoming his alcoholism: "Was God trying to talk to me during this time? You bet. Funny thing is, I thought I could hide it from him the same way I was hiding it from my wife. I thought if I ignored those gentle tugs on my heart, he wouldn't notice what I was doing."

With our overeating, are we also trying to ignore it? Do we hope that God isn't really watching, that he doesn't care? How do you think a holy and just God will deal with this kind of sin?

Due to the alcoholism, the husband in *Beyond the Shadows* lost his job, had an accident, and almost ran over his son. He said: "Most folks would wonder why that wasn't enough to make me stop. It's hard to answer that question except to say the fire of my addiction was burning white hot in my belly by that time."

Is that where I am too? How much have I lost due to my overeating? How much have I given up? Yet—have those losses made me get a grip on my eating? The reality is that I sin because I get something out of it, even if it ruins my life. I sin because I want to. Sometimes it's only a serious consequence that will wake me up. It might be high blood pressure, a type 2 diabetes diagnosis, or a heart attack. Whatever has happened, or even if it hasn't happened yet, the time to repent is now. I can't wait for the consequences to get worse.

Father, please bring me to a place of true awareness of my sin. And when I do repent, please meet me where I am and help me find the way out. Amen.

by Nancy

November 8

So if the Son sets you free, you will be free indeed.
John 8:36

How many of us dream of freedom? Oh, sure I think I'm free. I can hop in the car whenever I want. I can speak freely without worrying about being killed for it. But do I have the freedom to lay down the fork? Do I have the freedom to say no to the potato chips? Evidently I don't, or I wouldn't be here in this place of obesity.

I long for the kind of freedom where I don't have to worry about making wrong choices. I long for the freedom where if I don't need an extra helping, I won't have it. What keeps me from that freedom? What's holding me in bondage to the food?

I wish I had the answer for everyone. Many people would like to lay it on Satan, but we give that fallen angel far too much credit in our lives. Instead, I believe it's something different for everyone. There is no pat answer. It's something I need to ask God about, something I need to let him reveal to me.

God does promise me freedom. It's for that freedom that he died. The more I talk to him, the more I read his word, the more I can truly see what is holding me in bondage. He wants to set me free from obesity. He wants to set me free from "stinkin' thinkin'."

He longs for me to live in righteousness. But it's up to me. He won't force anyone to sit down with him today. He won't force anyone to search within. So, the longer I keep running from him, the less freedom I will have.

Father, show me what to do to become free. Tell me what will work for me, personally, even if it wouldn't work for someone else. Guide me in the way you want me to go. In Jesus' name, amen.

by Nancy

November 9

Be joyful in hope, patient in affliction, faithful in prayer.
Romans 12:12

Let us then approach God's throne of grace with confidence, so that we may receive mercy and find grace to help us in our time of need.
Hebrews 4:16

What I notice by not eating to cover up my feelings is that I feel things more intensely. Not all the time, but some of the time. In other words, I'm not just one big walking hurt, thanks be to God, but once I stopped stuffing my feelings with food, I finally felt a lot of the negative emotions I've been trying to avoid all these years. I've learned to work them out and sometimes wait them out, without eating over them.

I've often heard the saying, "Turn it over to God." I understand now that real recovery from compulsive overeating comes in making and keeping a daily connection with God. When I truly practice that connection through meditation on God's word and through prayer, then the food doesn't call to me as it did in the past, no matter what I'm feeling.

In the past, I wasn't a very good prayer warrior, and I still have to consciously work at it. God is good about reminding me, but I'm not always good about hearing or obeying when he calls me to pray. I do better, though, the more I listen and the more I practice. I know that God honors my efforts, and he answers my prayers when I ask according to his will. And it is *always* his will that I refrain from compulsively overeating.

Father, thank you for teaching me to pray, for leading me into fellowship with you every day. Help me to know and do your will today. Amen.

by Debbie

November 10

Finally, brothers and sisters, whatever is true, whatever is noble, whatever is right, whatever is pure, whatever is lovely, whatever is admirable —if anything is excellent or praiseworthy—think about such things.
Philippians 4:8

He has removed our sins as far from us as the east is from the west.
Psalm 103:12 NLT

God puts it plainly. I am to think on the good.

How many times do I see myself and then concentrate on the bad? I'm so ugly. I'm so fat. I'm a complete and utter failure. When I find myself thinking those things, I look at that scripture and realize I'm not doing as God has asked.

God says he created me. God says he loves me. God says that when I believed in his Son, he put my sins as far away from me as the east is from the west. That I am now a child of God. Jesus died for *me*. For *you*. I am that important. You are that important.

I love to sing the song, "Come Bless the Lord." Instead of letting words of condemnation get me down, I will lift up my hands and bless the Lord. I'll give God the glory for the victories in my life. I'll lift up my hands and declare the truth: I am a child of the Most High God! I'll never forget these words:

I praise you because I am fearfully and wonderfully made;
your works are wonderful, I know that full well.
Psalm 139:14

Father, help me to know the truth of your word, what it says about me. Not just with my mind, but deep in my spirit. In Jesus' name, amen.

by Nancy

November 11

Rejoice in the Lord always. I will say it again: Rejoice!
Philippians 4:4

A song that was stuck in my head recently is the one with the lyrics: "I've got the joy joy joy joy down in my heart." I've been thinking about when I have "the joy" in my heart. How do I behave? Where are my thoughts? Do I feel motivated, or am I just existing? When I'm having a good day, I'm more motivated to do what I need to do in this life. I want to make better changes. I want to succeed. On other days, when I'm not joyful, I just want to survive the next twenty-four hours.

I had a friend who was an awesome prayer warrior. We prayed together all the time. We would get into such fits of laughter we would roll on the floor. Our kids thought we were bonkers, but we didn't care. We had such joy in the Lord. If we can find joy in the Lord, we'll also find joy in the things around us.

When I was younger, I knew someone who was never without a smile. It's amazing how I don't remember many people from those days, but I remember her. She didn't always have things to smile about. She had cancer; she was on chemo. Yet there was that smile. Her joy was in the Lord; it wasn't in the circumstances around her.

It's so important to have time with Jesus every day. I admit that I'm still working on doing that, because some days I'm in survival mode. But I pray that each morning will begin a joy-filled day in the Lord. Like my laughing friend. Like the woman who always smiled.

Father, fill us till we're over-full with your joy. Help us to look at you, not at the circumstances around us. In Jesus' name, amen.

by Nancy

November 12

Not that we are competent in ourselves to claim anything for ourselves, but our competence comes from God.
2 Corinthians 3:5

If you're like me, there are days when you look back and wonder where the time went. Days when you feel like you didn't accomplish anything. But are those days really wasted?

I wrote in my journal about one such day (Note: I live with my aging mother and my disabled adult daughter):

Today was another day that in the past I might call wasted. But was it really? I read my devotional in the morning. I did my core-strengthening exercises for ten minutes. I washed dishes this morning so Mom wouldn't have to. I picked up COVID masks (made by a fellow church member) and delivered them to the neighbors. I cleaned my daughter's table fan for her, because Mom was horrified at how dusty it was. I cooked dinner for all of us. I made a to-do list for tomorrow. I also spent some time on Facebook, but during the pandemic it's the one way we can socialize without meeting in person, so was it a waste of time?

It's important to keep perspective. It helps to review the day and understand that just because I haven't checked off all the items on my to-do list doesn't mean that I haven't done anything worthwhile. I need to be open to God's leading, to doing what he brings into my life to do, and to do it with willingness and gratitude that I'm there to serve when service is needed. Even if it's not what I originally expected or intended to do.

Thank you, Father, for bringing those things into my life that you want me to do. Keep me open to what your will is for me each day. In Jesus' name, amen.

by Debbie

November 13

The royal daughter is all glorious within the palace;
Her clothing is woven with gold. She shall be brought
to the King in robes of many colors; The virgins, her
companions who follow her, shall be brought to You.
With gladness and rejoicing they shall be brought;
They shall enter the King's palace.
Psalm 45:13–15 NKJV

Do I see myself as royalty? If not, then am I seeing God as a King? And me as his child?

Sometimes I have to connect the dots. Sometimes I look at the heap of the mess that's in my life and don't connect myself with the One I need to stay connected to. The One who can help me make sense out of the mess.

I tend to see what's right in front of my face and not look within. It's hard to realize all that the Bible says I am. All that Jesus says I am. If I could only tap into that, then I believe I would see myself in a whole new light.

I am royalty. I am a child of the King.

Today I will enter into the King's palace. I'll take a stand about who I am. Because I'm a child of the King, I can live a life of fullness. A life of contentment. A life of peace.

And a life of knowing that I don't need food to satisfy me. Because what I need is right there in the palace, where I'm already welcome. Where I'm part of the royal family!

Father, you have adopted me into your family. Because you are the King, I am a daughter of the King. Help me to see myself the way you intend me to be—a member of your royal household. Help me see the truth of that. In Jesus' name, amen.

by Nancy

November 14

You have searched me, Lord, and you know me. You know when I sit and when I rise; you perceive my thoughts from afar.
Psalm 139:1–2

Therefore encourage one another and build each other up.
1 Thessalonians 5:11

Once, at Christmas party, I looked at the ten people seated around the table, and I thanked God that I have such good friends. Friends who were willing to carpool with me and my two girls to the town where the party was held. I was just so thankful that I could go and laugh and be with people who love me for who I am. But in this weight-loss journey I have become more aware of self-perception. As I was writing in my weight-loss journal one night, I told the Lord that I don't recognize myself. I don't like what I have become. I want my old self back. I want the freedom that I felt back then.

As I wrote, I was looking in the mirror, and the tears were streaming down my face. What is it that has caused this edifice that I call a body to groan under layers of unneeded fat? I am buried deep beneath the weight of the rubble. I need to dig myself out. I want to dig myself out.

It was then I was reminded of those friends. They can see the real me under all that rubble. They can see me.

So can the Lord. And he loves me anyway.

Father, thank you that you are the Lord who sees me and loves me anyway. Thank you for friends who do the same. Guide me and direct me as I seek your way out of my misery and despair, even when I have caused it myself. Help me to become the person you always meant me to be. In Jesus' name, amen.

by Nancy

November 15

Then Jesus told his disciples a parable to show them that they should always pray and not give up.
Luke 18:1

Rejoice always, pray continually, give thanks in all circumstances; for this is God's will for you in Christ Jesus.
1 Thessalonians 5:16–18

Something I read in one of my daily devotionals is P.U.S.H., which stands for Pray Until Something Happens. It's something I want to always remember to live by.

How I feel I need to apply it is this: When I feel the need to eat when I've already had enough when I want to eat at night when I should be done for the day, when I'm tempted to eat something I shouldn't, that's the time to P.U.S.H. through. To pray until something happens, until I'm willing to stop eating, until I'm willing to wait until I feel full, until the desire to eat passes, and until the temptation is lifted.

Every time I have actually done that—prayed until something happened—the desire to eat has passed. Disappeared entirely. I survived the momentary urge and discomfort without giving in.

Instead of my default position, which has always been the opposite, to turn to the food first, I pray that "P.U.S.H." will help me remember to turn to God first.

Father, when I need it most, please bring P.U.S.H. to my mind so that I'll always remember to pray until something happens, to pray until you lift my desire to overeat. In Jesus' name, amen.

by Debbie

November 16

There is a way that appears to be right, but in the end it leads to death.
Proverbs 14:12

We demolish arguments and every pretension that sets itself up against the knowledge of God, and we take captive every thought to make it obedient to Christ.
2 Corinthians 10:5

The truth is that life throws us curves. And sometimes I wonder if life is all mind games. I believe that some of it certainly is.

For example, I used to be a big soda pop fanatic. At one time, I was drinking six to eight cans a day. I could not get enough of that stuff. So I got to wondering, what was it about pop? Besides the taste, what had me so attached to it? I realize that in part it was because when I was little we didn't have it around the house much, so when I became an adult and could choose my own food and drink, it's something I could have. So I wanted it. No matter what, I wanted it!

How many things that I eat or drink do I choose only because I now have the so-called freedom to choose to have it? It doesn't matter how unhealthy it is. It doesn't matter what it costs. If I was denied it as a child, then I want it—now!

That's how my mind will play games with me. It's one of Satan's biggest tools. So I must allow God to show me what's behind the wrong thinking and make sure I take my thoughts captive, and bring my thinking into alignment with God's thinking.

Father, when my mind is full of wrong thinking, please show me, correct me, and bring my thoughts into alignment with yours. In Jesus' name, amen.

by Nancy

November 17

Because the Sovereign Lord helps me, I will not be disgraced. Therefore have I set my face like flint, and I know I will not be put to shame.
Isaiah 50:7

At some point I realized it's not a sin to be overweight. It's the stuff that goes with it that's the sin. We must repent of the gluttony and the selfishness that leads to overeating.

Why is it selfishness? When we choose to overeat and our health suffers, we aren't thinking about our families, about the people who depend on us. If something happened to me, I wouldn't want my kids to say, "I wish she would have lost the weight." It takes self-study and evaluation to understand why you're overweight. Sometimes we don't understand it ourselves, and we must ask God to show us. And then spend time with God working through it. We must then be willing to do what God asks us to do.

Yet once we have repented, we can no longer hang our heads in shame. God has forgiven us. I always struggled with that old saying, "You made your bed, now lie in it." I felt that if I made the problem, why would God want to help me? My mom often told me that I'm too hard on myself. That's true. No one needs to beat me up, because I do fine on my own.

But is that really how God wants us to be? God is saying, "Yes, you made the mess, but I want to help you through this." He wants to show me how to fix the problem. He has not given up on me. He does not want me to walk around in shame. I need to accept His forgiveness. I need to accept his help.

Father, help me not to hang my head in shame anymore. Help me remember that you forgive ALL my sins, not just some of them. In Jesus' name, amen.

by Nancy

November 18

Give thanks to the Lord, for he is good; his love endures forever.
Psalm 107:1

I know what it is to be in need, and I know what it is to have plenty. I have learned the secret of being content in any and every situation, whether well fed or hungry, whether living in plenty or in want.
Philippians 4:12

When I start thinking my life is really bad, I'm often reminded of people who are worse off than me. I think God does that to help me keep things in perspective.

I can pray and ask God to remind me of the things I have to be grateful for, and it helps even more to write it all down. It's called a gratitude list. It's impossible to be thankful and to simultaneously feel sorry for yourself; gratitude *quickly* wipes away self-pity.

One of the wonderful things that has happened over the years of walking with Christ is the sense of being content in all circumstances. In the past couple of years, I have experienced some financial uncertainty, but in the midst of that, God has met every need. What that has done is build my trust in him.

That doesn't mean I don't have dreams; I still do. But as I work toward achieving them, I can still be content where I am right now, today. That is in part because Jesus lives in me, and in part it's the result of walking in recovery. It's a gift.

Thank you, Jesus, for giving me the gift of the Holy Spirit, who gives me a sense of God's presence every day. When I feel that, I can feel contentment and joy and peace in every circumstance, because I know you love me with an everlasting love. Thank you for that. Amen.

by Debbie

November 19

Then young women will dance and be glad, young men and old as well. I will turn their mourning into gladness; I will give them comfort and joy instead of sorrow.
Jeremiah 31:13

David was dancing before the Lord with all his might . . . bringing up the ark of the Lord with shouts and the sound of trumpets.
2 Samuel 6:14–15

This last week God has had me thinking of joy, happiness, and dancing. Have you ever noticed that weight-loss programs often promote dancing? Dancing in your room. Just moving. We're supposed to keep moving. Yet there are times when the last thing I want to do is dance. There are so many pressures. So much stress. Or I'm too tired. But it's the very thing I find excuses not to do that will release happiness in me.

I have fibromyalgia, so there's not much exercise I can do without increasing my pain, but I can dance in my own home. I have no rhythm, but that has nothing to do with it. It's about doing something enjoyable. Releasing endorphins and having fun. I can put on dance-with-praise music and see how high I can soar with the Lord.

Father, some days the pain is so intense with the fibromyalgia that I can't even begin to think about wanting to dance. But I know that's what you want me to do. You want me to live free in the moment every now and then. To just soar with you. There is joy in the dance. So today, I'll take a little time to do a two-step with you. Please remind me when you want me to do it again. In Jesus' name, amen.

by Nancy

November 20

Look carefully then how you walk, not as unwise but as wise.
Ephesians 5:15 ESV

During the COVID-19 pandemic, I was taking part in a women's Bible study via Zoom, and before the ladies got started, there was some general sharing and banter. I listened to several ladies talk about foods they had brought into their homes that became problematic, especially being stuck at home so much. These are normal-weight women, people whom I would call "normal" eaters (as opposed to compulsive eaters like me). I was surprised to discover that they also have their food "weaknesses." They talked about sugary desserts or snacks high in fat and salt—some of the same things that are also problematic for me. The difference between them and me is that their response was to quickly recognize the problem and to make a decision not to bring those items home, to not keep them in the house anymore.

As a compulsive overeater, my past response was usually to buy *more*. To eat more of what I loved and craved and then inevitably overate. That makes me different mentally. It probably means I'm also different bodily, that my system has a different response to certain kinds of foods. Even so, I don't have any less responsibility than normal eaters to be wise about my food choices. In fact, I need to be *more* cognizant about what I put in my mouth, and I need to consciously follow God's leading in in my food choices. If I don't, I'll continue to be unwise and eat things that will springboard into overeating, resulting in poor health. The good news is that I have an advocate in God, who is always willing to listen and help, if I ask.

Father, give me your wisdom regarding my choice of foods. In Jesus' name, amen.

by Debbie

November 21

May the God of hope fill you with all joy and peace as you trust in him, so that you may overflow with hope by the power of the Holy Spirit.
Romans 15:13

If you're happy and you know it clap your hands.
If you're happy and you know it then your face will surely show it.
If you're happy and you know it, clap your hands.

Do you remember singing that as a child? We used to substitute the word "life" for "face." Does my life look happy? Someone once told me she loved to hear me laugh because I'm so sober all the time. That's not how I want to be seen. I'd rather be known as the life of the party. I want to have fun, to share my joy with friends and family. But can I show that when I am not really happy with myself?

I struggle with not being happy in my own skin. I want to get there someday. No matter what—at an ideal weight or not—we all need to be happy in our own skin. I often tell my kids to be content in the here and now. I should take my own advice. I can be happy at the weight I am right now within my life in Christ. That needs to come before everything else. But what does my life with Christ look like? Happy? Or down all the time?

If you're like me, you want to be happy where you are right now —but it has to be legitimate. There's a difference between faking it and being legit. I don't want to fake it. I want people to know that I'm legitimately happy in my life with the Lord.

Father, I'm clapping my hands. I choose at this moment to be joyful in you. I want my life to show it every day. Help me to see the joy in each day. Bring back the laughter. Let me be happy and truly know it. In Jesus' name, amen.

by Nancy

November 22

Because your love is better than life, my lips will glorify you.
I will be fully satisfied as with the richest of foods;
with singing lips my mouth will praise you.
Psalm 63:3,5

Why do I want more, Lord? Why isn't what I already had enough? What's missing inside me that leads me to think I need to eat to fill it up, even when I know my stomach is already full? What is it that I'm feeling—that I'm often unable to define or even understand—that makes me feel empty?

Am I feeling tired? Bored? Unhappy? Lonely? Angry? Frustrated? Helpless? Hopeless? Afraid? Something else? A lot of the time I don't even know! I've tried to fill it with everything else under the sun. Money. Recognition. Achievement. Status. Nice clothes. My dream car. Romance. Love. Children. Entertainment. Knowledge. Alcohol. Food.

Even as I'm asking, I find that the emptiness has lessened. It's going away. What a lesson that is! It means that when I turn to you instead of to food, I start to feel full again. Full of you. Full of love. Not empty anymore.

It's clear to me now that there's an empty place inside each of us that only God can fill. When I try to fill the part of my soul that's meant to be filled by God alone, I'm in reality committing idolatry. When I fill that place with fellowship with my Creator, I have ultimate fulfillment, because that's the reason I was made.

Father, keep me aware of you at all times. Make me aware that you are the only thing that fully satisfies my soul. Lead me to the place where my soul is refreshed, where my spirit is comforted, in you alone. In Jesus' name, amen.

by Debbie

November 23

Those who know your name trust in you, for
you, Lord, have never forsaken those who seek you.
Psalm 9:10

Trust can be a big word. It means "a firm belief in the reliability, truth, ability, or strength of someone or something." Sometimes people break our trust. Or they don't earn it. For me, trust is a deep thing. So much has happened in my life that I don't trust easily. And if someone loses my trust, it's hard to earn it back. We've all had someone let us down. Yet I start out by trusting everyone—that's what I expect, that they won't do things that hurt me. Then when they do—I have to step back and work through all those emotions.

God says, "Trust in me." Can I believe in God's reliability? Can I believe that he never wants to hurt me or forsake me? That's an easy answer: I trust God fully *with my life.* I trust that he will never do anything to hurt me, and he has never broken that trust. He has never let me down. Sometimes I wonder about unanswered prayers, but then I realize that throughout my life everything has turned out for good. Even when I don't understand, I trust that God knows what's best for me.

Do the people around me consider what's best for me when they make choices about how to treat me? Not always. God tells us to be careful, to make sure we're around people who want to help us on this journey, not people who want to sabotage or hurt us.

Trust that you can trust God! He is the only way.

Father, help me know that you always have my back, that I can put my full trust in you. You've always been here for me and will be, forever. In Jesus' name, amen.

by Nancy

November 24

Let the peace of Christ rule in your hearts.
Colossians 3:15

On disappointment: Don't immediately brush it off. Feel it first, and then it will leave you quicker. Here's the thing about broken glass: it needs to be acknowledged and swept up, so you don't step on it later.
Victoria Erickson

God made me to feel things: joy, sadness, love, hate, anger, compassion, disappointment, contentment. I've felt all of those things at one time or another. And I need to experience and feel my emotions as they happen so that I can deal with them, if necessary. If I don't acknowledge my emotions and give them to God, I may end up wallowing in them, letting anger become resentment or bitterness, for example, or letting disappointment become self-pity.

Yet in the past, anytime I was uncomfortable about something, I got an urge to comfort myself with food. Often, what made me uncomfortable was a negative emotion I was feeling. Even the mild ones made me want to eat.

Instead, I have learned to recognize that "this too shall pass." Whatever emotion I'm feeling is always temporary. If I understand that, then I don't have to follow the urge to reach for food as a way of comforting myself. Instead, I now have tools to deal with those feelings. Prayer is number one. If I turn to God, my Maker, the One who understands me best, he is always faithful to give me an answer and make a way out of my compulsion.

Father, when I get the urge to reach for the food, be quick to remind me that you are my Comforter and that I should always turn to you first. In Jesus' name, amen.

by Debbie

November 25

See, I am doing a new thing! Now it springs up; do you not perceive it? I am making a way in the wilderness and streams in the wasteland.
Isaiah 43:19

Oh, hallelujah! God says he is doing a new thing. Do I see it? I get so choked up thinking about just how much my Father loves me. How he wants so much better for me. He desires to see me break through my struggle with food. He wants to see me at the finish line, running through that banner, my hands in the air.

Oh, the celebration! Oh, the joy I will feel! And I can just see the Lord smiling big when he sees that I have broken through. That I have made it through the pain. That I have made it through the lessons that I had to learn so I could walk in freedom the rest of my days. He desires so much for me to have good things. He wants to run through that banner with me. Can I picture it? Can I see it? Can I feel it?

I know we all have it in us to succeed. We all can find the willingness to fight and win. I just can't wait to taste and see that it is oh so good! Can we all raise a hallelujah?! We are victorious. Even in reading this you are victorious. That shows that you desire it. You want it. You're researching. You're looking to see what God has for you to guide you to freedom. Count each step forward as a victory. No matter how big or small it is, it *is* a victory.

Father, please help me to see victory in myself. Help me believe that I can break through. I will see the finish line, and I will be celebrating with you and with all my loved ones. Oh, the freedom that I'll feel when I'm released from this bondage. Thank you, Lord, for desiring that for me also. In Jesus' precious name, amen.

by Nancy

November 26

The Lord does not look at the things people look at. People look at the outward appearance, but the Lord looks at the heart.
1 Samuel 16:7

God chose the lowly things of this world and the despised things—and the things that are not—to nullify the things that are, so that no one may boast before him.
1 Corinthians 1:28–29

I recently read a devotional about how often things look impressive and then when you experience the real thing, it's often a letdown. Not so great after all. The person with the beautiful face ends up being cruel. That thing you thought would bring you happiness ends up hurting you instead. The flip side of that coin is how often the things of God don't seem remarkable at all. Sometimes, they're even repellent. They often seem difficult, uncomfortable, or dangerous. Then, when you examine them closely, you find their true value. Those things become more precious than gold. As valuable as jewels. Objects of true beauty. The job you lost opened up the way for you to start the business you always wanted. That handsome guy who dumped you meant you were available when the love of your life finally came into the picture. That serious illness you went through brought you to the point of salvation.

I've discovered that God can use my difficulty in losing and keeping off the weight, my struggles with overeating, to help me grow up and learn things he desperately wants to teach me. I just have to be willing to see things in a new way. His way.

Father, open my eyes to see things the way you want me to see them. Help me to see the value in the very things I struggle with daily. In Jesus' name, amen.

by Debbie

November 27

You were taught, with regard to your former way of life,
to put off your old self, which is being corrupted by its deceitful desires;
to be made new in the attitude of your minds; and to put on the new self,
created to be like God in true righteousness and holiness.
Ephesians 4:22–24

What is a habit? The dictionary says a habit is a recurrent, often unconscious pattern of behavior that is acquired through frequent repetition.

How many times have I grabbed a cookie unconsciously and then afterwards realized what I've done? Isn't it amazing how we never quite notice it until after the fact? Could that be Satan trying to get the upper hand?

I was thinking about worrying. Is worrying a habit? I think so. It is recurrent. It's often unconscious. Do we worry about how we will get the extra weight off? Do we worry about what the scale will say? Do we worry that we will not be forgiven for the thousandth time?

Today, I'll take time to ask forgiveness for all those bites that I took unconsciously. I'll ask God to open my eyes to those times, to make me aware of what I'm doing.

And then I'll ask for forgiveness for all that unnecessary worry. Really, where does worry get me? Will it get me another pound down before my next weigh-in? Or will it get me another cookie in the mouth?

Father, help me become aware of ingrained habits and the things I'm doing right now that could become destructive. Then help me turn to you to break those habits—whether it's worrying or eating or something else—that you want me to change. Help me now in my great weakness. In Jesus' name, amen.

by Nancy

November 28

You will keep in perfect peace those whose minds
are steadfast, because they trust in you.
Isaiah 26:3

"I'm ugly. I'm just a fat sow. I may as well give up. I'll always be like this. I'm the cellulite queen. I'm not worthy of anyone's love. I deserve what I get. I'm gross-looking. I'm a slob. I'm nothing but a pig. I'm an ugly cow. I deserve to be treated badly."

Does any of that sound familiar? I know they are some of the things I've said to myself. I would guess many of you have also put yourself down a time or two.

But putting myself down doesn't make the weight come off. It doesn't draw people in or make them want to spend time with me. It won't make me healthy. And most of all, putting myself down grieves the Lord.

I don't believe that God made me fat. I'll take the credit for that one. But God made me who I am. So, even though I have put extra pounds on, I'm still putting down the person God created. Who am I to knock what God created and said was good? Remember that we're made in his image. When we put ourselves down, does that mean we're putting him down also?

Does he want me to love the fat? No. He wants me healthy and able to do the work he has for me to do. Putting myself down won't accomplish that. It only hurts me and the Lord.

Father, help me to keep my mind steadfast on you. Give me an accurate picture of how you view me, and help me not to say bad things about myself. Help me to see myself as the valued and loved daughter of the King that I am. In Jesus' name, amen.

by Nancy

November 29

The Lord replied, "My Presence will go with you, and I will give you rest."
Exodus 33:14

I read a meme on Facebook that said, "Taking time to be with God is the best place to find strength." It reminded me of a portion of the twelve steps (step eleven) that says, "Sought through prayer and meditation to improve our conscious contact with God." And that reminded me that I cannot do this thing called life without God's power. Actually, that's not quite right. I can do it, so can anyone. I just can't do it *well.*

And I really would like to do this thing called life well. That means I must actively seek out God, take the time to pray, and stay in his presence. And whenever I have done that, I have found his strength, his wisdom, his guidance, and his comfort. That makes me so grateful. When I think about God's presence with me throughout the day, throughout my life, I experience such gratitude . . . I think, *Thank you, Jesus. Thank you for your love, your goodness, your lovingkindness toward me. Thank you for your provision.*

The great thing about prayer is that it's just talking. Talking to Jesus like a friend. Telling him my feelings, my sorrows, my joys. Arguing with him occasionally. And if I'm honest, asking a lot of questions: Why is this taking so long? Why do I keep failing at this? What do you want me to do now? Is this the right thing to do? Yet, if I'm completely honest, most of my prayers are some form of, "Help me!" And that is exactly where he wants us. He wants us to depend on him. To be able to do that, I have to talk to him first.

Father, let me never forget my need to talk to you daily. Help me develop a discipline of prayer so I can get closer to you. In Jesus' name, amen.

by Debbie

November 30

But one thing I do: Forgetting what is behind
and straining toward what is ahead.
Philippians 3:13

But Lot's wife looked back, and she became a pillar of salt.
Genesis 19:26

God tells us not to look back. As I continue on this weight-loss journey, I can see why. There are so many days that are uplifting. Then there are those that are downright disheartening.

You know those gains and losses. You just never know if the scale will be kind—or not. How many times, as I take that step slowly up onto the scale (it's a big step, you know) do I take in a deep breath and pray that it will be good news?

It's what I do with each day that matters. If the scale shows a gain, then I look to the future. I work a bit harder. I keep my eyes on the prize ahead of me. I don't want to turn to salt, so no looking back.

This is a whole new life for me. The very basics must change for this to work. If I can't have junk food in the house, what will I snack on? When I'm hurting, sad, or stressed, what will I do instead of eating? When I can't grab a bottle of soda pop, what can I grab? Exercise—what's that? Should I keep driving around looking for a closer parking spot or choose to walk farther to get into the store?

Each moment of my day is a decision. Will my decisions be wise today?

Father, keep me aware of what's in front of me. Help me choose that water, the exercise, and going to you instead of food. Help me choose life today! In Jesus' name, amen.

by Nancy

Cry of Our Hearts

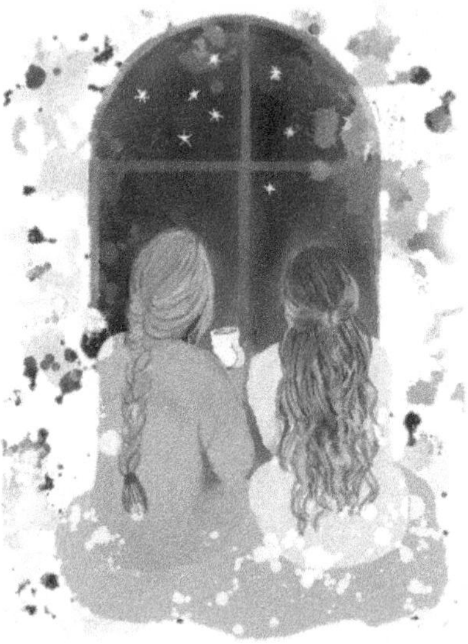

SERVICE and SUPPORT

We learn to help and support others.

In this section, we also share stories about how we came to faith in Christ and the wonderful ways God has worked in our lives.

Cry of Our Hearts

December 1

The pleasantness of a friend springs from their heartfelt advice.
Proverbs 27:9

This was written by our dear friend, Kathy, who has since passed on:

I'm so glad that we are all here at this appointed time. I've been so blessed that you're all here and love me no matter what. I'm so glad that I can count on your prayers and that we can keep each other lifted up. I know this is a special place, knew it as soon as I joined!

It seems like no matter what it is that we need, we find it when we come to our sisters in Christ, pour out our hearts, ask for help, or just want to encourage one another, perhaps even by having a good time bantering back and forth.

God's evidence in our lives isn't just seen by those around us at home, work, church, etc., but is evident to those of us who are joined together through Christ. It also comes in the shape of having someone cross my mind and know that you need prayer at that time. It comes from the sharing of God's Word and the insights we've received from it. It comes in the evidence of the love that is sent abroad throughout the world, sisters over the airwaves connecting through some tiny fiber, unexplainable, but we use it nevertheless!

I'm so very proud to call each one of you my sister. Short, tall, thick, thin, to me, you are more beautiful than you'll ever know. For God lets us see through our hearts, and all I see is his beauty in each of you.

Jesus, make us willing to minister to one another in the same kind of love our sister had for us. And keep her safe in your arms until the day when we can be with her again and share in her joy at being with you. Amen.

by Kathy

December 2

The way of fools seems right to them, but the wise listen to advice.
Proverbs 12:15

Part of my recovery from compulsive overeating involves reading recovery literature every morning. Today, I noticed something I must have underlined the last time I read it: *Cravings are not commands.* I decided to see what else I've underlined over the years. I realized that these sayings—written by those with years of experience overcoming compulsive eating—have often helped me profoundly:

- *Think. Pray. Act.*
- *Overeating enslaved me.*
- *Half measures get half results.*
- *If I disagree with God, guess who's wrong?*
- *Only the disease tells me that poison is a treat.*
- *Humility means . . . I realize there is a God, and it isn't me.*
- *Being willing to do something and wanting to do it are not the same.*
- *Each day I need to renew my commitment to abstinence from compulsive eating.*
- *The search for connection to a Higher Power is the "hole" I tried to fill with food.*
- *We cannot think ourselves into good action, but we can act ourselves into good thinking.*
- *When the pain of where I am is worse than the fear of where I'm going, then I'll welcome change.*

It's so important to learn from the wisdom of others!

Father, thank you for the support I receive from reading what others have written about what really works to overcome addiction. In Jesus' name, amen.

by Debbie

December 3

Now a man who was lame from birth was being carried to the temple gate called Beautiful, where he was put every day to beg from those going into the temple courts. When he saw Peter and John about to enter, he asked them for money. Peter looked straight at him, as did John. Then Peter said, "Look at us!" So the man gave them his attention, expecting to get something from them. Then Peter said, "Silver or gold I do not have, but what I do have I give you. In the name of Jesus Christ of Nazareth, walk." Taking him by the right hand, he helped him up, and instantly the man's feet and ankles became strong. He jumped to his feet and began to walk. Then he went with them into the temple courts, walking and jumping, and praising God.
Acts 3:2–8

Part of what keeps me out of the food and in recovery from compulsive overeating is giving service. Like Peter in the passage above, I don't have a lot of money to give, but I can give what I do have. I have time, I have at least a little wisdom, I may have some insight or a perspective about a problem that a person can't see herself. I may only be able to give an encouraging word.

But how many times has someone said something to you that he or she may have long forgotten, but you never have? I have many examples of those times in my own life. There are a few times when I've been reminded of things I said to people that I don't remember that made some positive difference to them.

The idea is to do what I can with what I have to give. It may not seem like much, but to someone, it may mean everything.

Father, most of the time it seems I have so little to give, but what I do have, let me give it freely. Bless those little gifts in ways I can't even imagine, so that I may contribute some good to this scary, often brutal world. In Jesus' name, amen.

by Debbie

December 4

For you formed my inward parts; you knitted me together in my mother's womb. I praise you, for I am fearfully and wonderfully made. Wonderful are your works; my soul knows it very well. My frame was not hidden from you, when I was being made in secret, intricately woven in the depths of the earth. Your eyes saw my unformed substance; in your book were written, every one of them, the days that were formed for me, when as yet there was none of them.
Psalm 139:13–16 ESV

Do you ever get together with friends and feel "off"? Like you're the fattest one in the group and they're judging you? Some friends and I had been invited to a Christmas party at a different church. We thought it was for supper. When we got there, it was all fancy desserts. When you're a bit heavier you sometimes think that if you take something that's considered fattening everyone will be watching and thinking "She doesn't need that." I was with the best group of friends. There was not one word spoken about my weight. We laughed and had the best time. And I realized that night that they loved me for who I am.

I once wrote in my journal that I don't recognize myself anymore. I don't like what I've become. I want my old self back. I want the freedom I felt back when I was thin. I look in the mirror, and I'm crying. I look in the mirror and wonder who I am. I'm buried deep beneath the rubble of the weight. I need to dig myself out. But my friends can see who I am beneath that rubble. So does God. God says I'm fearfully and wonderfully made. Can I choose to see myself as he does?

Father, help me to see myself as my friends see me, as you see me, as your child, a child much beloved by a wonderful Father. In Jesus' name, amen.

by Nancy

December 5

In the same way, let your light shine before others, that they may see your good deeds and glorify your Father in heaven.
Matthew 5:16

There is a prevailing view in our culture that a person's religion is a private matter and that one ought not interfere with it. As a result, I have let fear sometimes keep me from doing God's will, let it keep me from telling others about the Good News and our hope in Christ. Fear *and* selfishness.

Yet as Christians we aren't called to live to the standard of our culture, but to God's standard. I don't know how much time I have left on earth, but I pray that God will help me to fulfill whatever mission he has left for me to do.

One thing I can do right now is decide to give service where I can. Helping other people actually helps me too. It helps me stay out of selfishness, and being focused on others keeps me grateful for the blessings God has provided in my own life.

Specifically, if I can help others learn what I've learned about overcoming my food addiction, by talking about my mistakes and by talking about what has worked for me, it in turn will help me to continue in my abstinence from compulsive overeating.

Father, sometimes I just need your encouragement. I need you to help me get beyond my fears so that I can reach out to others when they need help from someone "with skin on." Please give me the willingness to continue to serve you and others. Please give me the time, health, and energy to turn my life around and serve you to the best of my ability. In Jesus' name, amen.

by Debbie

December 6

"Because he loves me," says the Lord, "I will rescue him; I will protect him, for he acknowledges my name. He will call on me, and I will answer him; I will be with him in trouble, I will deliver him and honor him. With long life I will satisfy him and show him my salvation."
Psalm 91:14–16

Every day I read things that help me in my recovery from compulsive overeating and sugar addiction. One of them is the devotional *Voices of Recovery*. Today's entry really spoke to me:

Even after more than five years in this program, food thoughts still pop into my mind when I feel stressed, frustrated, or depressed. Although I would love to have complete freedom from such thoughts, I'm learning to accept that I have the mind of a compulsive overeater, a mind that automatically associates feelings of discomfort with the siren song of food. . . . no matter how strong my desire to eat may be, it's never the food that I really want; therefore, eating won't make me feel better. If I am upset and craving food, I really need to connect with my Higher Power, to spend some quiet time by myself, or to talk to a caring friend. Thus, recovery has taught me that even though I may think like a compulsive overeater, I don't have to act like one.

Food thoughts still come to me when I'm unhappy or frustrated. Sometimes they happen when I'm afraid or full of worry. Food is my "go-to" for comfort, and I don't always realize that's what I'm doing. But God has made a way out. If I remember to turn to him instead of to food, if I ask for help, he is always faithful to answer me in the very moment of my need.

Father, in my lowest moments, thank you for being my salvation. Help me when I turn to you in the midst of my weakness. In Jesus' name, amen.

by Debbie

December 7

My dear brothers and sisters, if someone among you wanders away from the truth and is brought back, you can be sure that whoever brings the sinner back from wandering will save that person from death and bring about the forgiveness of many sins.
James 5:19–20 NLT

As I was driving the other day, I noticed how I look down the road at where I'm going. I don't look right in front of the car. I tried it once, and it wasn't a good experience. If I had kept it up, I wouldn't have been able to see traffic coming until the last moment. The path toward God's truth is like that. I have to keep my eyes on it and on what God has promised.

Sometimes, if I only look at what's right in front of me, I won't make it. If I can stay focused on what's coming, then I can keep going toward the ultimate reward. I can achieve good health. Joy. Peace. I can know I'm walking in God's will. I can reach a place where the sin of overeating no longer has a hold on me.

One of the things I can do is make sure I'm not doing this alone. I need to confess my bad and good times to people who understand this struggle. We need to be able to lift each other up. We need to go after each other and help those around us to quit wandering away from God in this area. We need each other—to rescue one other from destruction.

Father, you want us to help one another. When I'm strong, show me where I can help someone else. When I'm weak, please let there be someone there who can pick me up from where I've fallen. When I take my eyes off the destination down the road, put someone near who can show me the right way to go again. And let me do the same for my sisters and brothers when they need me. In Jesus' name, amen.

by Nancy

December 8

Greater love has no one than this: to lay down one's life for one's friends.
John 15:13

I admire that scripture. From a distance. When I see a movie hero sacrifice his or her life for others, I admire what the hero has done. (There are so many examples! *Deep Impact*, *Independence Day*, *Lord of the Rings: The Fellowship of the Ring*, *Star Trek: The Wrath of Kahn*, *Star Wars: The Last Jedi*, *Terminator 2: Judgment Day* . . . .)

I just don't want to be the one who has to do it. I'm willing to bet that's true of most of us. But in real life we're in good company, because it was even true of Jesus. The night before he sacrificed himself on the cross for the sins of the world, he prayed, "My Father, if it is possible, may this cup be taken from me. Yet not as I will, but as you will."

I don't want to feel the pain. I don't want to be tortured as Jesus was. And I have plans. I'd like to live a full life. My survival instinct is strong and God-given. But God has called me, as a believer, to walk in his footsteps. I may not ever have to die for someone, but I am called to sacrifice my daily life, my self-will, to help the people around me.

That's the ultimate kind of service. The ultimate kind of giving. Can I do it perfectly? No. I'm human, and I have human needs. I'm limited in so many ways. But I can give the things I have to give: my time, my knowledge, my abilities, my talents. My friendship. And I can work on giving it willingly rather than grudgingly. And if I'm ever called on to give up my very life—and I pray that I'm not—I hope that I'll have the strength.

Father, strengthen me as I seek to give friendship and support to others. Help me give service according to your will. In Jesus' name, amen.

by Debbie

December 9

Each of you should use whatever gift you have received to serve others,
as faithful stewards of God's grace in its various forms.
1 Peter 4:10

I watched a news story about a lady who needed to lose two hundred pounds; she had already lost a hundred. She was doing it by eating healthy food that "tastes like dirt." She was willing to eat it to lose the weight. But what made the biggest impression on me were her friends and family, who had rallied around her.

About a hundred people had offered their support, starting with three friends who wanted to help. They made a calendar, and for each level of weight she lost, a name was written on that date. The people agreed to work on whatever area of life they needed to, health, fitness, smoking, etc. So, when she hit that name on the calendar, then as of that day the person had to quit smoking, etc. I thought, *What awesome friends!* And, *How important it is that we have a support system!*

We need to be rooting each other on. We need people surrounding and helping us through each step of our weight-loss journey. That's why I'm so thankful to have a group of online friends to turn to. They have been a lifeline for me.

But we also need to make sure we have support up close and personal. If you feel that you have no one around to help you, seek people out. I know someone who got her coworkers to work toward a weight-loss goal together. Another friend attends Overeaters Anonymous. Others go to Weight Watchers and TOPS. We all need a little help from our friends. (I love that song.)

Father, help me find the right group who will support me as I try to live for you with my food and my life. And help me be a support to others. Amen

by Nancy

December 10

Do not work for food that spoils, but for food that endures to eternal life, which the Son of Man will give you. For on him God the Father has placed his seal of approval.
John 6:27

"Nothing tastes as good as abstinence feels." That's something I've heard sometimes, and what it refers to are the rewards that come from a lifestyle that's different from what I could have ever imagined: abstinence from compulsive eating.

I never pictured a life without eating sugar, a life in which I weigh, measure, and count my food (because I no longer trust myself to recognize normal portions). In the past, a certain kind of eating (sugar, salt, fat, and minimal vegetables) ruled my life, and whenever I tried some other way of eating, a diet designed specifically to lose weight, I always failed. Food became an idol, a god in my life, and I bowed down to it every day, not realizing that's what I was doing. I had always failed at diets before, because diets "cleaned up the food" temporarily but didn't address what caused me to turn to it for comfort.

Now, it's Jesus who is my idol, which is entirely appropriate. He said he is the Bread of Life, the Living Water, the Light. He said he is the Way, the Truth, and the Life. He said that he is God. When I turn to him for spiritual sustenance and direction, I can fill that void with him instead of the false god of food.

And he is enough.

Father, thank you for your sacrifice, for taking my punishment, for your willingness to lay down your life for me. The depth and breadth of your love is astounding, astonishing, and amazing. Help me to honor that love with my life. In Jesus' name, Amen.

by Debbie

December 11

Out of the same mouth come praise and cursing. My brothers and sisters, this should not be. Can both fresh water and saltwater flow from the same spring? My brothers and sisters, can a fig tree bear olives, or a grapevine bear figs? Neither can a salt spring produce fresh water.
James 3:10–12

I have discussed with people about how bad it seems with talk. I wonder if anyone can find anything nice to say anymore? Yet our words can affect people for days, months, even years.

Something happened one Sunday that just ruined my day. It had me upset for several days. It was such a petty thing. It wasn't even worth bringing up to me. What was said showed a spirit of meanness, and it sure didn't show any of God's grace.

I've heard it said many times that we just need more grace for one other. Isn't it better to look past the pettiness and just show some grace toward a fellow, frail, weak human being? Someone who is just like us? My mom used to say, "If you cannot say anything nice, then say nothing at all." I bet yours did too.

We all need uplifting. We all need encouragement. We don't need nitpicking and other words that hurt people. We don't need to tell people everything they're doing wrong. Who's to say you're right and they're wrong, anyway?

Rather, be encouraging. Tell them what they're doing right.

Father, help me to forgive mean people. I know often they are hurting too, and that's why they say mean things. And, Lord, keep my heart pure and my words uplifting. Don't let me ever do the same thing to someone else that has hurt me so much. Instead of tearing someone down, help me to lift them up. Help me to be supportive and encouraging. In Jesus' name, amen.

by Nancy

December 12

In that day you will say: "I will praise you, Lord. Although you were angry with me, your anger has turned away and you have comforted me. Surely God is my salvation; I will trust and not be afraid. The Lord, the Lord himself, is my strength and my defense; he has become my salvation." With joy you will draw water from the wells of salvation.
Isaiah 12:1–3

I was reading Jonathan Cahn's *The Book of Mysteries*; he wrote that in the passage above, the Hebrew word for salvation is *Yeshua.* That's the Hebrew name of Jesus, which literally means "Is Salvation." So it reads: "the wells of *yeshua*." The imagery of this passage is so beautiful. It makes me think of Jesus describing himself as providing Living Water so that we'll never thirst again. I live in the Pacific Northwest where water is everywhere: in Puget Sound, in lakes, rivers, and creeks, and on the tops of mountains as snow. It falls from the sky—frequently. But I've also lived in Southern California, a "Mediterranean" climate, so I know what dry means. In that climate, in the time Yeshua walked the earth, water was salvation, and its abundance was cause for joy.

Today, I want to walk up and drink from the wells of Yeshua, drink the Living Water so that I'll never thirst again. I can do that by believing that Jesus is my Salvation. That he came and paid the price for my sins so that when my life is over, I can have a home with him forever. Anyone can drink from the same well and receive the same living water. All you have to do is ask.

Yeshua, thank you for paying the price for my sins. Thank you for being my Redeemer, Deliverer, and Savior. Thank you for doing what I could not—for taking away God's anger toward the injustices of my sin so that I could one day walk into heaven and be welcomed with open arms. In Jesus' name, amen.

by Debbie

December 13

Out of the same mouth come praise and cursing. My brothers and sisters, this should not be. Can both fresh water and saltwater flow from the same spring? My brothers and sisters, can a fig tree bear olives, or a grapevine bear figs? Neither can a salt spring produce fresh water.
James 3:10–12

Something happened to someone I love dearly. A choice was made about what to say about it. A choice *could have been made* to uplift and encourage. Instead, the choice was to lecture. To not even acknowledge the good part of it all.

A choice was made to focus on what someone *thought* was the most important thing. But who was that person to say, to know, what was most important?

I wonder if the choice had been made to uplift, to encourage, how much differently the result would have been. I bet the recipient of the tongue-lashing would have instead wanted to be all he could be for the other person. I bet he would have wanted to work hard for the person and make him proud.

Instead, I suspect he went home with an attitude of "Why try? I tried hard, and it wasn't good enough."

God says there is power in the tongue. Power to kill or uplift. Proverbs 18:21 says: *The tongue has the power of life and death.*

If we make up our minds to choose only to encourage people in their Christian walk, or even just as they're walking through life, how different things could be!

Father, direct my words as well as my actions. If I've been speaking negativity into someone's life, show me so that I can stop. Make the words of my mouth and the meditations of my heart acceptable in your sight. In Jesus' name, amen.

by Nancy

December 14

God's love has been poured out into our hearts
through the Holy Spirit, who has been given to us.
Romans 5:5

Indeed, under the law almost everything is purified with blood,
and without the shedding of blood there is no forgiveness of sins.
Hebrews 9:22

When I gave my heart to Christ, he put his own Spirit within me. I still don't understand how that works—I may never understand it fully. I'm just glad it's true.

What it means is that while I'm still alive here on Earth, God is working within me to make me a better person—to make me more like himself. I don't understand that, either! I'm not sure why he left us so imperfect, but he did. Maybe in part because it would cause us to have to lean on him. Maybe because it would cause us to have to continue to learn the lessons he has for us.

We're all familiar with filters—we use them on our smartphones on our photos, and now we use them on social media or in meeting apps, like Zoom or Skype. Even in our imperfection, God looks at us as if looking through a filter, which is the blood of Jesus Christ. I'm so glad of that, because it means I can walk with God without the weight of guilt from my sin coming between us. My heart is full of gratitude for his love and forgiveness, because it means I can go to God as a much-beloved daughter and ask him to meet my needs. And sometimes even my wants, as long as those wants are aligned with his will.

Father, thank you for making the way to heaven by sending your Son to die in my place so that you could fully forgive my sins. In Jesus' name amen.

by Debbie

December 15

I was raised in a Christian home, but when I was nine I had a dream that Jesus was rounding up people to go to heaven. I knew he wouldn't pick me! The next Sunday, I went forward at our church altar call. I didn't have much sin to confess, but I knew I was a sinner and needed to accept Jesus as my Savior if I wanted to go to heaven.

By the time I was thirty-four, I had encountered a lot of pain and religious abuse and was not interested in biblical things, even though I was married to a preacher! One day while I was driving, a song came on the radio: "His Mercy Endures Forever" by Carman. It described to a "T" what I was going through. I looked to my right and "conveniently" there was a Christian bookstore! I bought the cassette and listened to that song all the way home, crying and asking God to forgive my cold heart and bring me back to him:

Maybe you've left your walk on the shelf, and you've lost some ground. You've fallen again and you feel so condemned, till it's got you down. If your sin has dimmed the Spirit's light, there's forgiveness through the blood of Christ, he'll restore your torn and shattered life. That's the reason I can say, that I will confess that my spirit's at rest, 'cause his mercy endures forever. Though troubles won't cease, yet my mind is at peace, 'cause his mercy endures forever.

At the time, my life was a shattered and broken "hot mess." I still have times when I doubt, but I know that is just Satan trying to stop me from living a successful and triumphant Christian life. If he can keep us confused, then we are worthless to the Kingdom of God. I don't want to be worthless; instead, as Bill Shivers of Brian Free & Assurance, sings: "I want to leave with nothing left," having used it all for God.

Father, thank you that your mercy endures forever. In Jesus' name, amen.

by Willie

December 16

Do not be afraid, for I am with you; I will bring your children from the east and gather you from the west.
Isaiah 43:5

My grandmother was a devout Christian; she and my aunts took me to church when I was young. I got saved at twenty-two, but I strayed. At thirty-two, I'd been married and divorced. My ex-husband asked me to go to a revival. The preacher spoke against fortune-telling; I had been consulting mediums for years. I went to the altar and rededicated my life to Christ. I haven't been to a fortuneteller since. God also delivered me from alcoholism and smoking.

I couldn't tell you all that the Lord has done for me. Growing up, my cousin was raised with me like a sister. When she was ten, she received third-degree burns over 90 percent of her body; they said it would be a miracle if she lived. Prayer brought her through, and she is now in her sixties. When I was raising my kids, I was never without a job more than two days. Sometimes I didn't have much left, but the Lord always provided. When I had surgery a few years ago, I "coded" for nine minutes. I don't remember going to the hospital and nothing else until I woke up in ICU. The Lord brought me through that too. Over many years, my family drifted apart, but the Lord brought us back together, including my cousin and my son who was in prison. I'm not rich as far as money goes, but I'm rich in so many other ways. There's so much the Lord has done, and I believe that includes things I don't even know about. I'll never know what I would have gone through if it hadn't been for him. It's been a wonderful journey with the Lord.

Father, help me to continue to take life day by day, praising you for what you do and not letting what goes wrong get me down. In Jesus' name, amen.

by Audrey

December 17

Taste and see that the Lord is good.
Psalm 34:8

As a child I was afraid of my father's rage. Along with horrific beatings, there were words that replayed in my mind: *You are useless. Why were you ever born? I hate myself.* I also experienced sexual abuse by another relative. As a young teen I thought about suicide. By my late twenties, I was married and had two beautiful children, but life was terrible. I was depressed and turned to food for comfort, yet I was out of control. I couldn't fill the aching void inside my soul. One day I saw an ad for Overeaters Anonymous. At a meeting, I heard people share about a "Higher Power." I thought, *This is some whacky religious group.* So I left and didn't intend to go back. But a lady rang me, said she had missed me, and would love me to come again. I couldn't believe the power that unleashed!

I went to a second meeting, but made a smart comment when the lady spoke about God. I saw her falter, and it hit me that I was trying to destroy in her the very thing I desperately needed! I later poured out my heart to her about how I hated my father. She told me about the power of forgiveness; I scoffed. Yet those words hit home. Later, I kept saying the words "I forgive my father." I physically felt something lift off my shoulders. It was freaky. It was amazing. It was God! After many months of having words of life spoken to me, I asked Jesus into my heart. That was another amazing experience. I felt as if I were spinning around and around. After that, even colors seemed different. This was the beginning of my wonderful forty-year walk with my precious Jesus. He is real. He is alive!

Father, thank you for sending someone to tell me the truth about the gift of your Son, Jesus. Amen.

by Viv

December 18

Have I not commanded you? Be strong and courageous.
Do not be afraid; do not be discouraged, for the Lord
your God will be with you wherever you go.
Joshua 1:9

I believe God has always had a hand on my life, from birth. I'm a twin, so we were born early, and the doctor didn't give us a chance of making it. But God had other plans, even though in the 1950s they didn't have the technology they have today to take care of preemies.

I was a good kid and didn't run around. But I knew that there was more out there, and it wasn't what all the other kids were into. I always felt a pull to Jesus. When I was in my late teens, we went to a church camp. At the evening get-together someone talked about how Jesus was there for us. My parents were divorced, and I just felt lost. After the meeting, I gave my life to Jesus. Later, I was baptized in the Lake of the Ozarks. I felt like I belonged to him. That's not saying I was always innocent; I did some things I wasn't proud of, but I always came back to him.

Later, I started working at the University of Missouri and got involved with the Christian Campus House. My faith grew even stronger over the years, especially after I began going to a small church in Ashland, Missouri. I started going there when my children were small and they went to school there. Most everyone there knew me from when I was young. They became my new family! It's been many years ago, and I have been through many trials, but I will never forget that night I came to faith in Jesus!

Father, thank you for your faithfulness, for bringing me through trials and through all the wonderful experiences of my life. In Jesus' name, amen.

by Delores

December 19

In the world you will have tribulation. But
take heart; I have overcome the world.
John 16:33

Even though I walk through the valley of the shadow of death, I will fear
no evil, for you are with me; your rod and your staff, they comfort me.
Surely goodness and mercy shall follow me all the days of my life,
and I shall dwell in the house of the Lord forever.
Psalm 23:4,6

And all things, whatsoever ye shall ask in prayer, believing, ye shall receive.
Matthew 21:22 KJV

I grew up in church but didn't get saved until after marriage. I never really got into worldly stuff, but I was by no means perfect. I made plenty of bad decisions, but God saw fit to bless me anyway. He gave me a faithful husband who has never mistreated me and three great sons. They aren't perfect either and have made their own mistakes, but I am blessed to be their mother. I pray every day for them to make the right decisions.

The worst thing I've been through is the death of my daddy, but God has made a way for me to see him again in heaven, and it's very comforting to know that Daddy is no longer in pain. We have been through some other great trials in our family, and I may never understand why some things have happened, but through it all God has been good. I don't deserve everything he has done for me and given me, but I'm grateful for it all.

Father, thank you for providing the good as well as the bad, blessings as well as the trials I have learned from. In Jesus' name, amen.

by Stacey

December 20

For a day in your courts is better
than a thousand elsewhere.
Psalm 84:10

I grew up in a dysfunctional home; by age fourteen I was a drug addict. As an adult I dabbled in witchcraft, and my anxiety level was always high. My mom and stepdad invited me to a Bible study in the house of a Christian couple. I kept telling them no, but I had already started wondering, *Why are they always so dang happy?* At the same time, I was miserable, dying inside. I finally said I would come one time if they would promise not to ask again. They walked me from Genesis through Revelation and answered all my questions: *Oh, so God opened his mouth and the world was just here? How do dinosaurs and cavemen fit into this story? How does God justify starving children in Ethiopia?*

Yet they were so kind, and they had an answer for everything. At the end they asked, "Do you want to ask Jesus to be Lord of your life, put away your sin, and begin fresh tonight?" I was saying to myself, *No God would ever love me. You have no idea what I've done.* But I said, "Okay," and the power of God came over me. I saw a black vapor leave me, and I started taking big gasps of air. I said, "I can breathe! I'm not anxious!" When I came home, my physical appearance had changed so much that my husband noticed. A little later I took boxes of occult books, tarot cards, and rock music and burned it all. I immediately quit doing drugs, stopped drinking alcohol, and quit smoking. I began going to church. I felt a sense of peace, and my extreme paranoia and anxiety left. I knew that Jesus Christ was alive. When I think of what God did, it's immensely humbling. I don't know if he could have gotten my attention any other way.

Father, thank you for the miracle of your saving grace and mercy. Amen.

by Sue

December 21

And you shall know the truth, and the truth shall make you free.
John 8:32

I grew up going to church every time the doors were open, but that church was very legalistic, and I don't ever remember them saying we need to have a personal relationship with Christ. Because my husband also didn't feel comfortable at that church, we started attending The Christian Missionary and Alliance church. One morning at a ladies coffee hour, a lady spoke about how a lot of people are going to miss heaven by a foot—the space between your head and your heart.

In 1990, I was at my aunt's funeral talking to my cousin's husband. Though I had no such plans, I told him I was going to be baptized. That night I also had a dream about being baptized, and I realized I wasn't saved, that there was no connection between my head and my heart. I believed, and I did get baptized that spring, and my life has never been the same. It hasn't always been easy, but I feel free.

I had the privilege of leading both of my parents to Christ. For a long time, my mom and I didn't have the best of relationships. I was always trying to please her and never could, but eventually she started coming around. In the last seven years of her life, we had a much better relationship. My aging father had Parkinson's disease. One night he kept on saying, "They're not going to let me in," and I knew he meant heaven. I said, "None of us are good enough, but you remember that Jesus did die on the cross for us. Do you want to have peace and know you're going to be with Jesus?" I told him how, he prayed, and he never again said he wasn't good enough.

Jesus, thank you that your sacrifice on the cross has made us all free. Amen.

by Ria

December 22

He is risen. You are paid for. You are immortal now. He won't be long now anyway. The water of your baptism sealed it. The bread of his Body feeds it. Don't wallow in the muck with those who have no hope.
The Mad Christian (revfisk.com)

I grew up in a Roman Catholic family in a predominantly Roman Catholic small town. Any questions about God I had were well answered, though as a child and teen I wasn't interested in knowing more about my faith or growing in it. When our parish priest was diagnosed with cancer, he gave several talks on death and dying that gave me great comfort in knowing of God's love for me, though it was also something I doubted when life was hard.

And there were hard things in my childhood. My first thoughts of killing myself happened in sixth grade. I found out later that there was a history of depression in my family and that my parents contemplated not having kids. The thought that my three siblings and I may not have ever been born made me appreciate my life more.

When my husband and I went through pre-marriage classes, I converted to his denomination. Those discussions with the pastor inspired me to do more reading about God. After the death of my father, I delved more into the promises of scripture and the Bible's historicity and veracity.

After the birth of our second son, I was diagnosed with postpartum rapid cycling bipolar disorder. With support, counseling, and medication I learned how to cope with anxiety and depression. Knowing that God did not promise me a smooth and easy life, but did promise to be with me through it all has been a comfort. And the support I have received from his people has been a blessing.

Father, thank you for always being with me in this present darkness. Amen.

by Staci

December 23

Therefore do not worry about tomorrow, for tomorrow will worry about itself. Each day has enough trouble of its own.
Matthew 6:34

I was fifteen when I became a Christian at a youth fellowship retreat, but I fell away from the Lord when I got married. My husband was not a good man. He wouldn't let me go to church and got mad if I even mentioned God. After our divorce, I went to church and rededicated my life to the Lord. I was single for about ten years, and one day I prayed to the Lord that if he wanted me to stay single that he would take away my desire to meet somebody. It was just two or three weeks later that I met Will, and that was a real answer to prayer. He's such a good man; I couldn't ask for a better husband.

I don't know how people can live life without the Lord. I know that he's always there, that I can always depend on him, and that he always cares. The night my mother passed away, I went home and lay on the bed, and on the radio I heard the song "I Can Only Imagine." At that moment, I knew that Mom was in heaven, and I just bawled. Every time I hear that song, I think of my mother.

The scripture that means the most to me is Matthew 6:34, because I always worry, but it tells me that though there's nothing I can do, the Lord is in control. That's true even now as I have aged and felt the effects of arthritis and having to recover from multiple surgeries. If it weren't for all the prayers of my family and friends, I don't know where I would be. It's been a real trial, but God has been there through it all.

Father, thank you for your presence through all the years of my life and for helping me to understand that I never need to worry. In Jesus' name, Amen.

by Patti

December 24

*Every good gift and every perfect gift is from above,
and cometh down from the Father of lights, with
whom is no variableness, neither shadow of turning.
James 1:17 KJV*

As I think about Christmas and the gifts that we give and receive, it makes me think about our Father in heaven. We want to give and bless people. How much more does he want to do that for us?

He has said in his word how much he wants to bless us. To bless me. Sometimes I think he means only in the material/financial realm. But he thinks in every realm. One is my health. He wants me to feel good. He wants me to be healthy. He desires me to live a long life. He'll help me accomplish that, because that is yet another gift he wants to give me. He'll also provide me with knowledge and wisdom about what to do to reach that goal. I just need to accept it, open it up, tear into it, and thank him.

I believe that with those gifts other gifts will come. Like joy and peace. I can also find happiness in everything around me. Sometimes I'm so weighed down I can't see the good right there around me. Yet as I shed the weight, my eyes will be opened to all the goodness out there.

But I have to accept that first gift from God. And I have to open it up and *see* all the goodness he has for me.

Father, I know that you have so many good gifts you want to give each of us. Help me to accept what you have for me, to open up each of your gifts, and to walk in all the goodness you have for me. Thank you, Jesus, for the ultimate gift, the gift of yourself. Amen.

by Nancy

December 25

For God so loved the world that he gave his one and only Son,
that whoever believes in him shall not perish but have eternal life.
For God did not send his Son into the world to condemn
the world, but to save the world through him.
John 3:16–17

What was the greatest service ever given to mankind? There's no question that it was the death of God's son Jesus on the cross. Before God created the universe, he existed as a complete being, one in essence but three in person. He knew that if the people he created were truly to be able to love him in return, he would have to create us with free will, which allowed for the possibility that we would choose to go our own way. To him, we were worth it.

So before the world had been created, before a single person had ever taken a breath, he devised a plan that would allow for free will but also, knowing that mankind would choose our own way, make a way back from brokenness to perfection.

His own perfection demanded perfect justice, and the price for anything less was spiritual death—separation from him. So God became flesh as Jesus of Nazareth. And when Jesus had paid for sin with his death, he said, "It is finished." And it was, once and for all. All we have to do is recognize the price that was paid and Who paid it. We first recognize our shortcomings, then acknowledge what Jesus did for us. Believe that he died and that he rose from the dead as a sign that it was all true. Through his death and resurrection, we have hope for restoration of a relationship with the God who loves us and, ultimately, the restoration of the entire creation.

Father, thank you for the gift of your Son, for making a way for all things to be restored to the perfect world you intended in the first place. Amen.

by Debbie

December 26

This is the confidence we have in approaching God: that if we ask anything according to his will, he hears us. And if we know that he hears us —whatever we ask—we know that we have what we asked of him.
1 John 5:14–15

One wet winter's day, my brother and I were traveling home from high school. The bus left the city at 4:00 p.m. and usually took about thirty minutes to get to our farm in the country. That day, my mother glanced at the clock at 4:00. She suddenly had a strong urge to pray for us, a God-prompt that wouldn't go away. This was before cell phones, so she couldn't contact us to find out why. She just knew she had to pray right then.

Shortly after 4:00, our bus was hit by a drunk driver, causing it to slide off the wet road and hit a power pole topped by a huge transformer, which broke and landed on top of our bus. Everyone onboard was too scared to move as waves of fireballs rolled off the roof. I was sure we were going to be burned. Yet power from the broken lines didn't affect the bus; it flowed instead down unbroken lines into a nearby house, blowing out all their electrical appliances.

Because of the risk of fire and electrocution, we lined up and jumped into a muddy ditch, then moved away and stood in the middle of a wet field—in case the bus blew up. But no one on the bus was hurt, not even a scratch. Another bus turned up and took us home, late but safe. When my worried mother heard what happened she understood why God had prompted her to pray. I believe her intercessory prayer saved our lives. So, now, when God prompts me to pray for someone, I do. I may never know why or what the outcome will be, but I do know that God hears our prayers.

Father, thank you for often telling me even when and what to pray. Amen.

by Marilyn

December 27

Your faithfulness continues throughout generations.
Psalm 119:90

When I was a teenager I made some bad choices; I thought I knew better than everyone else. But there were people praying: my mom, grandma, and oldest sister, who also invited me to her church events. I experienced some bullying in school, so I tried the rough way first. I married at sixteen, and my daughter was born a year later. She is my miracle.

In January of 1986 I went to my sister's church, where I gave my life to the Lord. A few years later I had a stillborn son. A few years after that my first husband and I divorced. I went through a lot in that marriage, but God was faithful. I met my current husband a year later. After that we went through two miscarriages, which was a low point in my life. I was told that I couldn't try to have more children, but I was able to adopt my husband's three children a few years later. Our lives revolved around church while the kids were growing up.

God has been faithful to me through it all; he never left my side even when I went through years of depression. I always felt it was my fault my unborn babies died, that it was my body that had killed them. But God gave my mom the right words to dig me out of that mindset. God never promised us an easy life, but he promised to be with us through it all. I'm living proof of that. Even through the drinking, drugs, loss of babies, divorce, depression, and health problems, I never felt abandoned. I'm so grateful for January 12, 1986, the day I turned it all over to him.

Father, I'm so grateful for your mercy and grace, even through the times I wasn't serving you. Thank you for my family who prayed for me. Amen.

by Nancy

December 28

"Sirs, what must I do to be saved?" They replied,
"Believe in the Lord Jesus, and you will be saved."
Acts 16:30–31

I was in sixth grade when the Gospel was first presented to me. I thank God for my middle school Sunday school teachers who laid it out for me and that it is simple enough for an eleven-year-old to understand. After hearing it, I went home, got on my knees, and asked Jesus to come into my life. I know now that I was immediately filled with the Holy Spirit. At the time, all I knew was that I felt a profound sense of God's presence and love.

Not long afterward, I was praying and asked God to have someone call me. While I was still on my knees, the phone rang; it was the person I wanted to speak to. It was in that way that God began to build my faith in him. I was a child praying a childish prayer, but in that moment, I knew God was real.

Becoming a believer didn't make me perfect. I still had plenty of flaws and a strong self-will. I've made a lot of mistakes in my life, and I have rebelled against God many times. But it began a relationship with a very patient God, One who never gave up on me, One who is still working daily to make me a better person.

That first-love feeling is quieter now, but it has never left me. I still turn to Jesus when life becomes overwhelming. He's who I turn to when I get that hungry-when-I'm-not-really-hungry feeling. It's his strength, his power, and his love that enables me not to eat. When I turn to him in my moment of need, he is enough.

Father, thank you for filling my heart with your love and presence all those years ago. Thank you for being there for me now, whenever I need you. In Jesus' name, amen.

by Debbie

December 29

He who has an ear, let him hear what the Spirit says to the churches. To the one who conquers I will grant to eat of the tree of life, which is in the paradise of God.
Revelation 2:7 ESV

I looked up the meaning of the word "life." This is what it says: "The condition that distinguishes animals and plants from inorganic matter, including the capacity for growth, reproduction, functional activity, and continual change preceding death."

That means our life is ever changing.

We are constantly growing.

I sometimes question why I haven't got a handle on a healthier way of eating. A healthier way of living.

But this verse gives me hope. It shows me that God will not give up on me. I can keep learning. I can keep growing. And I can keep changing day by day.

I don't need to give up hope. I don't need to feel that it's not worth it. We have been given a gift by our Father that someday we'll get to eat of the tree of life in paradise.

As the saying goes, "Just keep swimming!" I can and will make it! I *will* conquer this problem with the Lord's help and a little help from my friends.

Father, thank you for all your promises. I so appreciate that you understand that my life is on a constant learning curve. You don't give up on me, and you help me up when I fall. You wipe my "boo-boos" so that I can move forward. I love you, Lord, with my whole heart. In Jesus' name, amen.

by Nancy

December 30

Keep this Book of the Law always on your lips; meditate on it day and night, so that you may be careful to do everything written in it. Then you will be prosperous and successful.
Joshua 1:8

It's important to keep in mind what God has said in his word. To meditate on its truth. To remember. Something I've tried to put to heart comes from Ephesians Chapters 1 and 2, which tell me who I am as a believer and what Christ has done for me:

I have been adopted into God's family.
I have been created to do good works.
I have been marked with a seal.
I have been made alive in Christ.
I have been saved by grace through faith.
I have been brought near to God.
I have been seated in the heavenly realms with Christ.
I have been blessed with every spiritual blessing.
I am the praise of his glory.
I am a citizen of God's kingdom.
I am chosen.
I am forgiven.
I am redeemed.
I am included.
I am God's handiwork.
I am a member of God's household.
I am God's dwelling place.

Father, thank you for your word and for how it speaks truth into my very spirit, for how it guides me, uplifts me, and blesses me. In Jesus' name, amen.

by Debbie

December 31

The Lord bless you and keep you; the Lord make his face shine on you and be gracious to you; the Lord turn his face toward you and give you peace.
Numbers 6:24–26

Know therefore that the Lord your God is God; he is the faithful God, keeping his covenant of love to a thousand generations of those who love him and keep his commandments.
Deuteronomy 7:9

As I've been writing, I've also been listening to version after version of the worship song "The Blessing." This song debuted in March 2020 near the beginning of the COVID-19 pandemic and quickly went around the globe. I put together a YouTube playlist that has eighty-four versions of the song, mostly from "virtual" choirs from across the world in almost every language you can think of (and in several you probably didn't know existed).

I have a few favorites. The one from the Pacific Northwest, where I grew up. The one from the place where the song originated, Elevation Church. Surprisingly, one that's sung in Dutch. The New Zealand version. One from Puerto Rico. But my absolute favorite is *Ha Bracha*, in Hebrew, the language in which this blessing was first spoken over God's people more than three thousand years ago. So, on this last day of the year, I'd like to "speak" a blessing from the song lyrics on you and on your weight-loss journey that will go out with you into the new year:

May his presence go before you, and behind you and beside you,
All around you and within you, He is with you, He is with you,
In the morning, in the evening, in your coming and your going,
In your weeping and rejoicing, He is for you, He is for you. Amen.

by Debbie

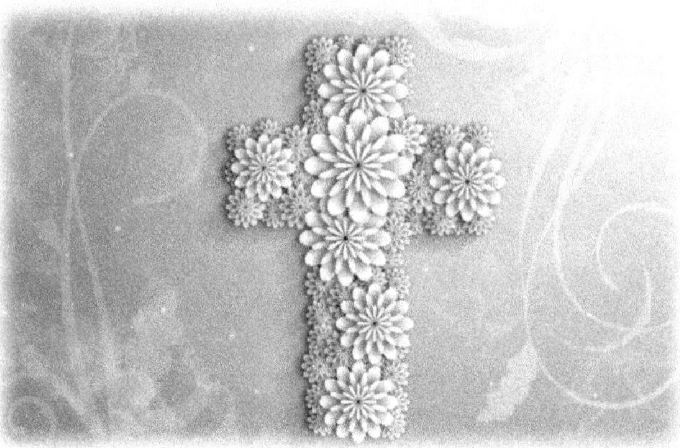

STATEMENT OF FAITH

WE BELIEVE

. . . the Bible is the inspired, infallible, true word of God.
. . . there is one God, eternally existent in three persons: Father, Son, and Holy Spirit.
. . . God is the creator of heaven and earth.
. . . mankind was created in the image of God and was originally free from sin. Being tempted by Satan, mankind fell from that original righteousness, causing all people to inherit a sinful nature.
. . . in the deity of the Lord Jesus Christ; he is the only Son of God, preexistent with God in eternity, was the prophesied Jewish Messiah, was born of a virgin, became fully human, and lived a sinless life.
. . . Jesus Christ died on the cross, was entombed, on the third day was bodily resurrected, and that he ascended to be seated at the right hand of the Father.
. . . at the moment of salvation, at the moment people repent and come to faith in Jesus Christ, believers experience spiritual regeneration by the Holy Spirit; they are born again.
. . . salvation comes through Jesus Christ alone and that it is offered freely to all who have faith in Jesus Christ.
. . . Jesus Christ will come again in glory to judge the living and the dead and that his kingdom will have no end.
. . . in the resurrection of both the saved and the lost at the end of the age; those who are saved to a resurrection of life and those who are lost to a resurrection of eternal separation from God.

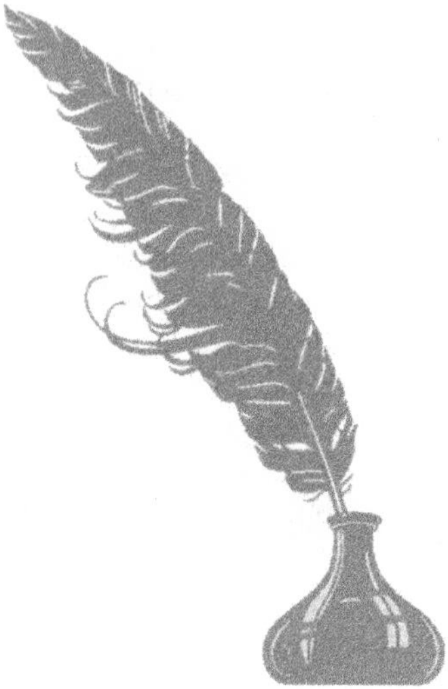

ABOUT THE AUTHORS

NANCY URBAN was born in St. Paul, Minnesota, but has been a small-town girl for most of her life. When she was quite young, her family moved to a farm outside of Alpha, Minnesota. Then when she was twelve, they moved into the small town of Alpha. She now lives in the small town of Welcome, Minnesota.

She attended Southwestern Technical College, studying to become a medical secretary and currently works as the office manager of her church. She is married and the mother of four children, all adults, and loves being a grandmother. She enjoys redecorating her house, working on crafts, and spending time with God and her family. She also finds it important to surround herself with supportive friends, with whom she loves to spend time—laughing and encouraging one another.

She says, "It is truly the cry of my heart to walk in God's ways at all times in every area of my life."

DEBBIE JACKSON grew up in Washington State in a small town north of Seattle but lived in Los Angeles for many years, which is where she raised her three children, now all adults. She recently returned to the Pacific Northwest.

She earned a BA in English from the University of Washington and then many years later earned a doctorate in psychology with an emphasis in organizational management and consulting from Phillips Graduate University in Chatsworth, California.

She has been a freelance editor and writer for many years and has recently started helping authors publish their books through her indie publishing venture, Áccent on Words Press. She is also currently an online-only adjunct instructor for Grand Canyon University, teaching four courses in human factors psychology, a specialty within the field of industrial/organizational psychology.

Debbie's favorite hobby is photography, though she's strictly an amateur and feels she has much more to learn. You can find some of her photos at pixabay.com by entering user:debannja in the search bar. She's also fiercely interested in Christian apologetics and writes a blog that includes some topics related to defending the Christian faith (beewisdom.wordpress.com).

She says, "It's the cry of my heart to always turn to God with everything in my life, especially as I seek to overcome my compulsion to overeat and, through this book, to pass along that knowledge and experience to others."

REFERENCES

Alcoholics Anonymous World Services (Ed.). (2013). *Alcoholics Anonymous* (4th ed.).

All Sons & Daughters. (2016). I Surrender [Song]. On *Poets & Saints*, Integrity Music

Anspaugh, D. (Director). (1993). *Rudy* [Film]. TriStar Pictures.

Bill P., Todd W., Sara S. (2005). *Drop the Rock: Removing Character Defects - Steps Six and Seven.* Hazelden.

Bolz, R., & Chewning, L. The Anchor Holds [Song]. Shepherd Boy Music, Word Music, LLC.

Brian Free & Assurance. (2017). Leave with Nothing Left [Song]. On *Beyond Amazed*, Daywind Records.

Isaacs, J, Rowland, M., & Shapiro, A. (Executive Producers). (2005). *Brat Camp* [TV series]. Shapiro/Grodner Productions.

Bunyan, J. (1678). *The Pilgrim's Progress.*

Cahn, J. (2018). *The Book of Mysteries.* Frontline.

Carman. (1984). His Mercy Endures Forever [Song]. On *Coming on Strong*, Myrrh.

Charmaine. (2002). Give Us Clean Hands [Song]. On *All About Jesus*, Elevate Records.

Delirious? (2011). Find Me in the River [Song]. On *You Never Let Go.* Integrity Music.

Dictionary.com. (n.d.). Follow. In *Dictionary.com.* Retrieved from https://www.dictionary.com/browse/follow

Dictionary.com. (n.d.). Life. In *Dictionary.com.* Retrieved from https://www.dictionary.com/browse/life

Emmerson, N. (Executive Producer). (2007). *Fat March.* [TV series]. Ricochet Television.

Francisco, D. (1993). Adam, Where Are You? [Song]. On *Forgiven*, Benson.

Green, K. (1990). My Eyes Are Dry [Song]. On *No Compromise*, Sparrow.

Hatcher, R. L. (2018). *Beyond the Shadows: A Novel.* RobinSong, Inc.

Hayford, J. (2003). *I'll Hold You in Heaven.* Chosen Books.

Hillsong. (2002). Amazing Love [Song]. On *Amazing Love*, Hillsong Music Australia.

Hummel, C. E. (1994). *Tyranny of the Urgent.* InterVarsity Press.

Jobe, K., Carnes, C., & Elevation Worship. (2020). The Blessing [Song]. On *Graves Into Gardens*, Sparrow.

Kent, C. (2007). *A New Kind of Normal.* W Pub Group.

Kohlenberger III, J.R. (2015). *The NIV Exhaustive Bible Concordance* (3rd ed). Zondervan Academic.

Lewis, C. S. (1965). *The Weight of Glory and Other Addresses.* Wm. B. Eerdmans.

Lewis, C. S. (1954). *The Horse and His Boy.* Geoffrey Bles.

Lewis, C. S. (1952). *Mere Christianity.* Geoffrey Bles.

Lewis, C. S. (1952). *The Voyage of the Dawn Treader.* Geoffrey Bles.

Maranatha Singers. (2012). Humble Thyself in the Sight of the Lord [Song]. On *Praise 3.* Calvary Chapel Music.

McBride, M. (2010). Anyway [Song]. On *The Essential Martina McBride.* RLG/Legacy

McReynolds, J. (2018). Make Room [Song]. On *Make Room*, eOne Music.

Mercy Me. (2001). I Can Only Imagine [Song]. On *Almost There*, INO Records.

Merriam-Webster. (n.d.). Disease. In *Merriam-Webster.com Dictionary.* Retrieved from https://www.merriam-webster.com/dictionary/disease

Merriam-Webster. (n.d.). Grace. In *Merriam-Webster.com Dictionary.* Retrieved from https://www.merriam-webster.com/dictionary/grace

Merriam-Webster. (n.d.). Integrity. In *Merriam-Webster.com Dictionary.* Retrieved from https://www.merriam-webster.com/dictionary/integrity

Merriam-Webster. (n.d.). Rebellion. In *Merriam-Webster.com Dictionary.* Retrieved from https://www.merriam-webster.com/dictionary/rebellion

Merriam-Webster. (n.d.). Repent. In *Merriam-Webster.com Dictionary.* Retrieved from https://www.merriam-webster.com/dictionary/repent

Meyers, N. (Director). (2000). *What Women Want* [Film]. Paramount.

Moore, B. (2007). *Breaking Free: Discover the Victory of Total Surrender.* B&H Books.

Overeaters Anonymous. (2002). *Voices of Recovery.*

Oxford Dictionaries. (n.d.). Responsible. In *Oxford Dictionaries.* Google.com

Reiner, R. (Director). (1987). *The Princess Bride* [Film]. Act III Communications.

Riso, R. (1992). You Prepare a Table [Song]. On *Scripture Memory Songs: Spiritual Warfare.* Integrity Music.

Schram, R. E. *The Living Last Supper: A Dramatic Musical Experience for Holy Week.* The Lorenz Corp.

Shirer, P. (2021). *Elijah - Bible Study Book: Faith and Fire.* Lifeway Press.

The Mad Christian. (n.d.). *Are You Mad?* https://revfisk.com.

Tolkien, J. R. R. (1954). *The Lord of the Rings.* Allen & Unwin.

Warren, R. (2002). *The Purpose-Drive Life.* Zondervan.

All images used in the book or on the cover are either created by the author/editor and therefore covered by U.S. and international copyright laws or are copyright-free. Images from pixabay.com were created by the following users: Nika Akin, Gerd Altmann, Mochamad Arief, Lorraine Cormier, Hannah Edgman, Graphics Ninja, Jeff Jacobs, Gordon Johnson, Alexandra Koch, Barbara A. Lane, messersrach, ractapopulous, Luciana Silva, and stux. Thank you for your creative and beautiful artwork!

All scriptures quoted in this book were found on the Bible Gateway website, www.biblegateway.com, and where no translation is noted are from the New International Version (NIV), with some excerpts from (where noted) the Contemporary English Version (CEV), the English Standard Version (ESV), the King James Version (KJV), the New American Standard Bible (NASB), the New Century Version (NCV), the New King James Version (NKJV), the New Living Translation (NLT), The Living Bible (TLB), The Message, and the World English Bible (WEB).

ÁCCENT ON WORDS PRESS

Thank you for reading this publication of Áccent on Words Press. To find out more about how you can also publish a book, contact the editor and publisher, Deborah Jackson, by e-mail via djackson@accentonwords.com.

For more information, visit accentonwords.com.

Áccent on Words Press

CPSIA information can be obtained
at www.ICGtesting.com
Printed in the USA
LVHW091541270821
696281LV00006B/73

9 781734 260526